Contents

Preface

Change has become a way of life as the twentieth century draws to an end. The modern population has grown used to regarding as temporary many aspects of the world of work that, in a more leisurely age, might have seemed fixed for a lifetime at least. Organisational reconfigurations and changes to policy and practice are accompanied by a hustle and bustle that draws attention, marking them out for good or ill; but there is the slower grind of macro-social change that proceeds almost imperceptibly. Even where separate factors are recorded along the way, the accumulated impact of apparently unrelated changes may intertwine and fuel a broader shift in values and working patterns that goes largely unremarked. However, as with each new generation, nurses today are aware that their daily practice and expectations are qualitatively different from the world views held by their parents and professional forebears.

This book represents an attempt to capture and hold up to scrutiny a number of different influences on nursing, that stem from the nature of the health care organisations in which nurses work and the views of society about nursing roles in the contemporary world. Underpinning the whole text lie two competing attitudes that may be adopted by nurses. First, nursing is perceived as a profession by many; they believe the key to quality improvement is to develop and promote that professionalism. Alternatively nursing may be viewed as a managed service; in that case the success of nursing as an occupation depends on its ability to colonise senior positions within the management hierarchy of health services. It is not easy to explore the relative influence or likely outcome of taking one view or the other, because in reality the two are closely intertwined. Indeed, the separate socialisation and organisation of nurses and managers into their different spheres of work leads to a dichotomy that may, itself, be false. In practice, nursing is often characterised in either way, but rarely as both; contradictions and dilemmas that arise tend to be viewed in oppositional terms of conflict.

This book attempts to explore the alternative viewpoints in a constructive way, so that nurses and health service managers might consider the potential benefits and probable difficulties in steering the occupation of nursing in either direction, or attempt to merge both into a different way of operating. Notwithstanding its title, there are three things that this book does not do:

(1) It does not tell nurses how to be managers
(2) It does not tell managers how to manage nurses
(3) It does not tell either nurses or managers how to create or cope with change.

These things are important, of course, and there is a wealth of literature about change in nursing elsewhere. There is remarkably little written about the other points, except in relation to specific projects or current policy topics – then ideas abound in print and in practice. There is no shortage of papers or people, either inside or outside the sphere of nursing, to advise on what nurses or managers 'should do' in a specific circumstance that warrants change. Nor is there a lack of guidance or influential opinion about leadership in nursing. However, there are curiously few books to guide aspiring managers as to the best way of managing nurses, and even fewer books to advise nurses wishing to enter the sphere of management. This supports our contention that the two spheres operate under relatively separate terms of reference and understanding; their different cultures lead to the use of what sociologists term 'alternative discourses', each locked into understanding the world only from their own particular perspective.

This can lead to an occasional sense of powerlessness or frustration, caused by the profusion and confusion of interdependent issues. This book aims to identify some of the most influential aspects of these interrelated systems and individual perspectives, then hold them up to critical scrutiny to unravel some of the taken-for-granted assumptions embedded within them. The intention of the editors was to allow equal attention to be given to the alternative viewpoints, seeking evidence from research to support or refute either case. It is probable that strong advocates of one attitude, whether managerialist or professionalist, will feel their own perspective has been under-represented or the other one afforded too much space. Also, some suggestions made in the chapters are quite radical, while others have been around for many years; these are still deemed sufficiently worthwhile to bear repeating, since planning for the future should always draw lessons from the past, maintaining the positive and discarding the negative as far as possible.

Nurses and their colleagues at all levels in the health care system are invited to use insights from the text, to question and search for further ideas, then map a course for the future, not so much as individuals but as members of a large and important occupational group. Positive action will result only if enough nurses agree about the most suitable way to achieve forward progress in their occupation, about how it contributes to human well-being and about its place in society. The book opens with a chapter that expands on the alternatives. Then, Section 2 offers two chapters that set the scene by exploring an ideal vision of nursing as a profession. In Section 3, the impact of managerialism on these ideals is explored in some depth, before moving to the concluding section which attempts to forge some links between the alternative, competing perspectives. At the start of each section, a brief commentary from the editors relates the chapter contents back to the main thrust of the debate.

Ian Norman
Sarah Cowley
London, 1999

List of Contributors

K. Louise Barriball, *BA, RGN*
Lecturer, Research in Nursing Section, Division of Nursing & Midwifery, King's College London, James Clerk Maxwell Building, Waterloo Road, London SE1 8WA.

Ann Bergen, *BA, MSc, RGN, DipN, DNCert, CertEd, DNT*
Visiting Research Fellow, Research in Nursing Section, Division of Nursing & Midwifery, King's College London, James Clerk Maxwell Building, Waterloo Road, London SE1 8WA.

Sarah Cowley, *BA, PhD, PGDE, RGN, RCNT, DipN, RHV, CPT, HVT*
Professor of Community Practice Development, Division of Nursing & Midwifery, King's College London, James Clerk Maxwell Building, Waterloo Road, London SE1 8WA.

Margaret Edwards, *BA, MSc, PGCE, RGN, RM, RHV, DNCert*
Lecturer, Research in Nursing Section, Division of Nursing & Midwifery, King's College London, James Clerk Maxwell Building, Waterloo Road, London SE1 8WA.

Joanne Fitzpatrick, *BSc, PhD, RGN*
Lecturer, Research in Nursing Section, Division of Nursing & Midwifery, King's College London, James Clerk Maxwell Building, Waterloo Road, London SE1 8WA.

Nicholas Hale, *BA, MSc, PGCEA, RN*
Senior Lecturer, Buckinghamshire Chilterns University College, Faculty of Health Studies, Gorlands Lane, Chalfont St Giles, Bucks HP8 4AD.

Kate Morrison, *BSc, MSc, RGN, NDN*
Nurse Practitioner, Broomwood Road Surgery, St Paul's Cray, Orpington, Kent.

Ian J. Norman, *BA, MSc, PhD, RMN, RNMH, RGN, RNT, DipAppSocStud, CQSW*
Professor of Nursing and Interdisciplinary Care, Division of Nursing & Midwifery, King's College London, James Clerk Maxwell Building, Waterloo Road, London SE1 8WA.

Sally Redfern, *BSc, PhD, RGN*
Professor of Nursing University of London and Director of Nursing Research Unit, King's College London, James Clerk Maxwell Building, Waterloo Road, London SE1 8WA.

Julia Roberts, *BA, MA, PhD, RGN, DipN, CertEd, RCNT*
Lecturer, Research in Nursing Section, Division of Nursing & Midwifery, King's College London, James Clerk Maxwell Building, Waterloo Road, London SE1 8WA.

John S.G. Wells, *BA, MSc, PGDipEd, RMN, RNT, RPN*
Lecturer, Centre for Mental Health Nursing, Waterford Institute of Technology, Waterford, Ireland.

Section 1
Setting the Scene

1 Nursing in a Managerial Age

Sarah Cowley

Introduction

This chapter explores the concepts of *professionalism* and of *managerialism* set out in the Preface, to consider how they relate to nursing in the modern rapidly changing world. A number of different influences on the occupation stem from the nature of the health care organisations in which nurses work and the views of society about nursing roles in the contemporary world. These influences give rise to two competing attitudes that may be adopted by nursing. One is that nursing is a profession at least in an emergent state; therefore efforts should be made to develop and promote that professionalism to enhance the quality of the service. The other view holds that nursing is a managed service; in this formulation, the key to nursing success lies in its ability to colonise senior positions within the management hierarchy of health services.

Themes raised in the discussion will be developed in the rest of the book, as subsequent chapters focus on different aspects that influence the organisation and practice of nursing. In the end, some conclusions will be drawn about how the occupation might cast itself in a new and different mould as the new millennium dawns.

Professionalism

The quest for nursing to be recognised as a profession dates back to at least the end of the nineteenth century (Hector 1973), which is hardly surprising given the importance afforded to professionalism within contemporary culture. Indeed, volumes have been written about the nature and sociology of professions. As Schön (1983) explains:

> 'The professions have become essential to the very functioning of our society. We conduct society's principal business through professionals specially trained to carry out that business . . . We look to professionals for the definition and solution of our problems and it is through them that we strive for social progress. In all of these functions, we honour what Everett Hughes has called the "professions" claim to extraordinary knowledge in matters of great social importance", and in return we grant the professional extraordinary rights and privileges. Hence, professional careers are among the most coveted and remunerative, and there are few occupations that have failed to seek out professional status'.
>
> (Schön 1983 pp. 3-4).

This notion of an extraordinary knowledge base is included in the classical view of what constitutes a 'profession'; Millerson (1964) lists the important characteristics. Professionals are held to use skills based on a specific (if not unique) theoretical knowledge base and to have education and training in these skills. Their competence needs to be assured by examination as a condition of entry to the profession. They use a code of conduct to ensure professional integrity and have a professional organisation; some commentators insist on a form of official regulation, such as state registration. Finally, professional status is associated with the performance of service for the public good. Friedson (1970) argues for a distinction between the ethos of professionalism and the formal reality of professional status; the authority to act autonomously in determining the nature of their practice is a pre-requisite for the latter.

These features have been much debated and the extent to which they can be considered 'definitive' of a profession, or even desirable for either society as a whole or nursing in particular, is open to question. Indeed, there are suggestions that professionalism is, itself, now a flawed and outdated concept that nurses should not adopt uncritically (Davies 1996a). This view will be explored as the knowledge base and professional regulation, autonomy in practice, and performance of a service for the public good are considered in relation to nursing.

Knowledge and regulation

Davies (1995) remarks on the professionalising zeal that has pertained through the history of nursing in the UK, starting with the protracted battles to establish a nursing register that was finally set up in 1921 after earlier legislation. At present some 640 000 people, slightly more than one per cent of the population, are registered across the 15 different categories regulated by the United Kingdom Central Council for Nursing, Midwifery and Health Visiting (UKCC).

Patterns of nursing regulation, education and training vary markedly from one country to another, although there are certain agreements, for example across the European Union, to enable workforce mobility across national boundaries. However, the very size and diversity of nursing militates against identification of the 'extraordinary knowledge' that could unify and distinguish it as a profession. That is not to deny the enormous strides made by the professionalising zealots in mapping the terrain and carrying out increasingly rigorous and impressive research to demonstrate the importance and effectiveness of nursing. It is, however, to acknowledge the continued existence of multiple different segments and expectations within nursing.

Melia (1984) drew attention to the distinct differences between the idealised world of nurse education, where student nurses learn a form of professional practice that is 'supposed' to happen, and the service sector in which the 'real work' is carried out. Recognising the existence of this segmentation and the theory–practice gap is neither new nor confined to nursing; the 'reality shock' experienced by newly qualified practitioners has been well documented (Kramer 1974). However, Melia's (1984) work graphically drew attention to the fact that student nurses subject to a transient apprenticeship during their training learned more about the 'student work' of fitting in and just passing through different settings as they gain experience, than about the 'nursing work' of patient care and workload management.

Another aspect of significance concerned the extent to which the 'untrained' (auxiliary nurses) instructed the 'unqualified' student nurses, casting doubts on the training system even as a form of apprenticeship (Melia 1984). Shortly after this research was reported, UK nurses officially secured full student status for half their formal period of preparation, along with an educational base in the university sector, albeit at 'sub-degree' level. However, funding for nurse education differs from that of other university students, remaining firmly under the control of the majority employer, the National Health Service (NHS) (Humphreys 1996). Furthermore, the shift created an immediate shortfall in the workforce that was largely replaced by non-professional nursing auxiliaries or assistants, raising questions about the nature of the 'extraordinary knowledge' required for professional nursing practice.

Such contradictions might undermine any reasonable nursing claim to have established a sufficiently differentiated or specific theoretical knowledge base to support their professional status. However, two different lines of defence might be proffered. First, Davies (1995) argues that the true work of nursing remains 'invisible' because of its gendered nature; citing Daniels (1987), she explains:

> 'The care that women give in the home and family setting is governed by values of love and spontaneity, is carried out in isolation from others, is bereft of validation by any source apart from the care recipient.... as far as women's paid work is concerned, the closer it is to the activities of nurturing, comforting, encouraging and facilitating interaction – features encompassed by the definition of caring given above – the more likely it is to be seen as natural or the expression of women's style in general.

(Davies 1995 p. 142)

Such analysis offers at least some support for the common view, taken up as a theme later in this book, that caring is a central and defining concept that influences nursing theory, nursing research, nursing practice and nursing education (Morse *et al.* 1994).

Regardless of its centrality, the idea that as ephemeral a concept as caring might form the core of a theoretical knowledge base for nursing seems doomed to fail, at least as long as professional knowledge is defined within the traditional model. Schön (1983) is a much cited critic of this traditional approach; he describes a looming crisis stemming from lost public confidence in the ability of professions to meet the greatest needs of society. The underlying reason for this, according to Schön, is because of a faulty view of what counts as 'knowledge' in the archetypal professions.

Orthodox definitions identify the major professions as those with unambiguous ends, a knowledge base that is firmly bounded, strictly scientific, standardised and located within a positivist epistemology. This 'technical rationality' viewpoint presumes that problems and desired ends can be known and predicted in advance. The 'real world' of practice tends to be unstable, shifting, unpredictable, unique and contradictory; for this a different form of knowledge that Schön calls 'professional artistry' is needed. Furthermore, he suggests that the problems of the greatest human concern lie, not in the 'high hard ground' of technical theory, but in the 'swampy lowlands' of everyday practice.

Nursing took great heart from this attack on the epistemological basis of traditional professional knowledge. There is now a vast and growing literature explaining, celebrating and researching various aspects of nursing expertise, intuition, artistry and professional judgement in terms that explicitly reject exclusive reliance on the positivist traditions of the former professional model. It is, however, noticeable that neither medicine nor management, both of which disciplines were used to illustrate practice examples within Schön's (1983) text (whereas nursing was not mentioned), have greeted the ideas with quite the same enthusiasm. There is, as well, increasing emphasis on evidence-based practice as a basis for informing health care commissioning and clinical governance; acceptable forms of evidence in this context continue to be drawn from a viewpoint of strict 'technical rationality', mainly in the form of randomised controlled trials. This returns to Friedson's (1970) view that the authority to act autonomously in determining the nature of their practice is a pre-requisite of professional status.

Autonomous practice

In a critique of nursing's determined 'professionalising project', Porter (1992) identifies two mechanisms by which the occupation has sought to gain authority and control over its own practice. He dismisses the development of hierarchies of nursing management as ineffective in this endeavour, partly because of the speed with which managers become divorced from the clinical work that they direct. Also, as power accrues to those higher up the management ladder, so the autonomy and status of clinicians is undermined still further.

The second strategy focuses on the position of these clinical practitioners, and attempts to enhance their autonomy in practice. Porter (1992) identifies medical dominance over nursing as the major obstacle to success in this approach, commenting on the remarkably limited attention paid to this relationship in the professionalising literature and concluding that:

'The construction of nursing as almost totally independent of, and separated from, medicine bears little resemblance to the day-to-day activities of most nurses, which involves considerable interaction with doctors.

(Porter 1992, p. 722)

It is a common organisational and public perception that nurses work only with individuals who are directly 'under medical orders' at the time, rendering nursing work necessarily subservient to medicine. The extent to which this is an essential aspect of the work and how much relationships conform merely to stereotypes expected within a highly 'gendered occupation' (Robinson 1991) is again significant. However, there is another issue. While Porter distinguishes between the idealised 'segment' of nurse professionalists, and a supposed real world of practice that bears little resemblance to the theoretical constructions developed by the former, he fails to acknowledge that the very diversity of nursing in so many different fields, levels of practice and methods of working is another form of segmentation.

The observation that nursing involves considerable interaction with doctors is particularly true for hospital nurses working within acute care settings, but (notwithstanding the alleged existence of primary care teams) less so in community situations. It becomes increasingly uncommon in situations where the recipients of nursing attention have either chronic, well-managed disorders or no immediate medical needs, despite having a nursing need. Everyday examples include the preventive and public health practice of health visitors, school and occupational health nurses, the continuing care of frail older people in nursing homes and nurses caring for people with learning disabilities. Innovations include nursing beds in rehabilitation or general hospital sites (Griffiths & Evans 1995), nurse-led Primary Care Act Pilot Sites (Cohen 1998) and the burgeoning nurse practitioner movement (Jordan 1994).

Melia (1987) recognised this huge diversity in practice, suggesting that the various nursing factions might be better regarded as a federation of craftworkers than as a unified profession. Conversely, Porter (1992) castigates proponents of so-called 'clinical elitism' for debarring second-level enrolled nurses (a practically based qualification that is no longer available) and even the unregistered from this occupational advancement. It is hard to know where he would draw the line given the even greater diversity among assistants who are paid from nursing budgets or who help nurses in a voluntary capacity. Again, a simplistic case might be made for hospital 'bedside workers' but it would be harder to decide whether to include as 'nurses' the link workers who interpret in well baby clinics, clerical assistants in school health work or home carers involved with bathing older people but employed by social services in the UK. An international stance would need to consider the huge range of often very skilled lay and village workers who operate within a nursing remit.

This debate, of course, invites two further comments. The first questions the nature and scope of nursing itself; it is at least possible that this is so broad and diverse that it would be quite impossible and probably undesirable to seek to professionalise all of it. A mother nursing a sick child, a spouse caring for a terminally ill partner or a school friend helping a child negotiate a ramp to the classroom in a wheelchair are all examples of non-professional 'nursing'; in these and many other instances care might be given with or without support from a professional nurse.

In a rather pejoratively phrased comparative analysis of lay caring and professional (nursing) caring, Kitson (1987) proposed that nursing was needed where a deficit or lack occurred in three aspects required to meet the demands of the recipient of care. These were a potential lack of commitment, of appropriate knowledge and skills or of ability to ensure the integrity and self-respect of the person in need of care; Kitson suggests that lay carers are particularly well-placed to ensure this third condition is met. A further interpretation might be to suppose that support, clinical supervision and caring for lay carers should, perhaps, be developed further as a nursing skill. This analysis draws attention again to caring as a central aspect of nursing, and also leads on to the second question, which concerns the nature of relationships between professionals and the public they serve.

Serving the public good

In a philosophical examination of the 'ideal' of professionalism, Moline (1986) hints at the significance of caring. He indicates that the spirit or attitude that the professional brings into a personal, fiduciary relationship is more important than any other aspect. However similar, knowledgeable or necessary the working practices of other occupational groups may be, he claims that the thing that distinguishes 'paradigm professions' (he gives the examples of medicine, law and the clergy) is the expectation that they will give supremacy to the needs of their client, above such considerations as profit, personal gain or the needs of the organisation that employs them. This suggestion might lead nurses to take heart from their allegiance to the caring ideal, offering examples of 'emotional labour' (Smith 1991) to demonstrate an indisputable altruism in serving the best interests of their particular public.

However, there are at least two difficulties with such an optimistic view. The first stems from the disputed nature of 'caring', of what exactly is meant by this and how it might benefit the recipients; in turn, this leads to lack of legitimacy for these aspects of the work. Paradoxically, health visitors interviewed by Cowley (1995a) attributed a lack of legitimacy for the supportive and caring aspects of their role to the fact that they were regarded as nurses. Doctors and health service managers were held to believe or insist that nurses carry out only definable tasks under medical direction.

The second criticism goes to the heart of the professional/client relationship, casting doubt on caring as a force for good. Malin and Teasdale (1991) make a direct link between the altruism implied in the caring relationship and the paternalism that stems from a relationship which assumes the professional expert should decide things in the best interests of the patient. Thus, caring may serve to disempower the recipients of care by promoting dependence rather than enabling them to develop their own autonomy, which is an essential requirement for health

(Rijke 1993). This critique has roots that reach back as far as Illich's (1976) famous polemic against medicine, in which he explicated the different forms of harm, or iatrogenesis, stemming from the increasing medicalisation of society. He identified cultural iatrogenesis, which destroys the potential of people to deal with their human weaknesses and vulnerability in a unique and personal way, as the most insidious and harmful of all.

Such concerns led Davies (1996b) to propose that nursing should take a lead in developing a new vision of professionalism. Nurses, she suggests, should not promote the old fashioned professional concepts of mastery of knowledge, unilateral decision-making (with the patient as dependent and colleagues deferential), autonomy and self-management, individual accountability, detachment and interchangeability of practitioners. Instead, they should develop a professionalism that promotes reflective practice, interdependent decision processes (patient as empowered and colleagues involved), supported practice, collective responsibility, engagement and specificity of practitioners' strengths.

However, Schön (1983) suggests that professionalism itself is in decline as a concept. He draws parallels between the way the industrial revolution changed for all time ideas about what it meant to reap the whole fruits of one's labour, and the anomie experienced by current professional workers whose work is continually subject, as Davies (1995) points out, to discontinuity and fragmentation:

> 'Fragmenting of nursing work into a series of tasks that can be treated as routines, in effect presents nursing as an activity that consists of a large core of "basic" tasks that can be accomplished (albeit under supervision) by people with little or no training, together with a number of more technical procedures that have to be the province of the trained.'

> (Davies 1995, p. 94)

Perhaps, then, nursing should look outside the professional arena altogether as a way of gaining control over the practice? The next section of this chapter will consider the potential of managerialism as a future model for nursing.

Managerialism

While professionalism celebrates the unique skills of individual practitioners in different practice fields, management is concerned with getting things done through others. The skill of the manager is, therefore, general rather than specific and the term encompasses a huge range of meaning. Two key aspects encapsulated in the wider discussions about managerialism are relevant for the purposes of this chapter. Organisational theory examines the way that the structures and hierarchies within systems affect the working practices and functions of people working within them. Sociological interest in management has focused both on the managers themselves as an advancing occupational group and on the technical and social control functions of the management process mediated through these organisational structures. Both aspects are relevant to contemporary nursing since they influence the views that nurses hold about their own self-image as either managers or professionals and how they feel about the organisation in which they work.

Change is a key focus for organisational theory. Attempts to develop flexible systems tend to be measured against descriptions of bureaucracy, which is the archetypal form of organisation first outlined by the sociologist Weber early in the twentieth century. Bureaucratic systems are characterised by subdivision of labour, specialisation of tasks, clearly defined rules and standards, impersonal processes and technical efficiency; work is delegated to subordinates and run with clear lines of authority from a single manager to each worker. These rational, hierarchical organisations have been likened to a well-oiled machine (Marsick 1987); it is assumed that they are directed primarily by their goals. Work is held to take place by direct cause–effect linkages while actions are thought to be governed by objective notions of reliability and predictability. They are arranged as a network of separate parts or tasks, all precisely designed to complement each other and to fit together to form a coherent whole. The system works like an assembly line and is eminently rational and efficient as long as the design remains fixed and unchanging.

Bureaucracies have long been roundly condemned mainly because of this inflexibility and their dehumanising tendency to treat people as parts of a machine (e.g., Schön 1971, Peters & Waterman 1982, Marsick 1987, Knowles 1990). However, just as it would be unreasonable to assume that the old-fashioned model of professionalism is the only one possible, so it would be improper to ignore the effect of modernising influences on managerial systems. Organisational theories have been the subject of debate, discussion and innovatory zeal as well. Parallels between the skills required to be a skilled health care professional and a 'real manager' in the modern sense of the word have been well stated (Iles 1997). Nurses may not wish, as Nyberg (1994) advises, to style themselves as 'professsnocrats' to celebrate their potential contribution to both managerial and clinical fields; but they may see the leadership potential in taking responsibility within organisational systems that are more innovative and flexible than the old-style bureaucracies.

Morgan and Ramirez (1983) suggest the metaphor of a hologram for guiding social change in organisations. A hologram is a laser-created photograph in which the whole is represented in all of the parts; it is not possible to separate out any single aspect or part of it. Morgan and Ramirez offer the brain as an example of a complex network and system that seems to operate on holographic principles. It is able to develop, learn and compensate naturally when parts are damaged or missing, or expand and adapt to new possibilities and potentials arising from the environment. Organisations might, perhaps, aim to emulate this capacity:

'How wonderful if our social institutions could possess this capacity. If we design them in accordance with holographic principles so that we could systematically attempt to build the functions necessary for the whole into the parts, then there is a chance that we could move toward this state of affairs – or at least make them much more responsive than they are now. The growing turbulence of the modern world suggests that it is vitally important to increase our ability to deal with the major changes that we create in our environment, and more importantly, to learn how we can manage relationships with our environment to avoid creating problems that we then have to solve.'

(Morgan & Ramirez 1983, p. 2)

The aim is to create systems that are able to learn from their own experience and to modify their structure and design to reflect what they have learned. There are three characteristics needed for a system based on holographic principles; these are requisite variety, minimum critical specification and substantial rationality. The principles will be explained and used to explore a modern managerial focus that parallels the key issues described under professionalism.

Requisite variety

The standard professional model emphasises the need for a separate, unique knowledge base for each discipline, which is problematic given the huge scope and diversity of nursing. However, complex organisations need just such a variety of skills and abilities to carry out their functions; Morgan and Ramirez (1983) emphasise the importance of building as much variety as possible into a system.

The old mechanistic model of management stresses the need for some 'spare parts' in the form of staff capable of undertaking particular tasks to cope with changes that might be anticipated, such as an additional demand or staff sickness. This approach depends on the idea of 'single loop learning' (Argyris & Schön 1978), which assumes that someone – perhaps a manager or someone important in the hierarchy – will identify any errors within the fixed system and correct them, because they are able to have a clear overview of the issues from 'on high'.

The expectation that people can be relied on to carry out only single, predictable functions does little to improve flexibility within a rapidly changing world; it also creates the task focus and fragmentation that offends so many nurses. Davies' (1995) complaint about the transience of the workforce and interchangeable use of qualified and unqualified nursing staff illustrates the tendency to treat nurses as parts of an overall health care machine. The approach ensures the work is subject to separation and fragmentation; the holistic nature of nursing is rendered 'invisible' and devalued within the system. This tendency is further increased as new technological equipment and effective medications simplify tasks that were once obviously 'complex' and therefore credible but had simultaneously allowed the close contact required for the invisible aspects of nursing to be carried out. Further, the inflexibility may create a significant value conflict for nurses, if they are forced to choose between meeting the needs of their patients or the goals of the organisation (Nyberg 1994).

Instead, Morgan and Ramirez (1983) suggest that the workers who are closest to the problems which arise in practice need both variety and control, in order to be able to deal with the diversity and unpredictability of practice. Rather than the mechanistic approach of seeking a 'redundancy of parts' in the organisational health care machine, a 'redundancy of skills' should be sought. This principle emphasises that for a system to cope with the problems and demands posed by the environment, variety equal to that found in the environment must be included within the system.

Such diversity may be found in complex teams of nurses who have different types or levels of skill, or in multi-disciplinary groupings. Integrated nursing teams within primary health care, for example, might encompass several distinct specialisms (Black & Hagel 1996), while single discipline teams incorporate several grades of nurse such as the one familiar at hospital ward level. Complex teams are exemplified by multi-disciplinary community mental health care teams (see e.g. Onyett *et al.* 1997), primary care teams (see e.g. Poulton 1994) or palliative care teams (see e.g. Hutchison *et al.* 1991). These arrangements encourage the valuing of specific skills for their contribution to the whole system rather than to a particular task; the assumption that the different skills are interdependent encourages sharing of responsibilities and development of individual practice (Marsick 1987).

Such multi-disciplinary and even multi-agency work is increasingly favoured in the 'care sector', which encompasses health and social care and the criminal justice services, statutory, private and voluntary services. A functional mapping exercise carried out to determine areas of shared interest and skill identified the nature of the caring relationship as a key function (Mitchell & Coats 1997); it was divided into three main aspects which were themselves then further sub-divided and enlarged: empowering users, enabling and intervening. The functional map was devised to inform the development of National Vocational Qualifications, but it serves additionally to demonstrate the shared abilities across a number of distinct disciplines.

Despite the wide range of shared functions, Mitchell and Coats (1997) stress the importance of recognising specialist expertise as the necessary core of professional identity and purpose. This ensures that managerial control remains within the specialist disciplines; in turn this helps avoid the interdisciplinary rivalries or alliances that counter the overall objectives of the agency. This echoes the requirement that the workers who are closest to the problem need to maintain both variety and control to respond flexibly to varying and unpredictable demands in practice, and potentially offers a more appealing system to nurses than one that emphasises the need for a unique, single knowledge base. However, control does not automatically accrue because variety exists; the wish for professional autonomy is considered next.

Minimum critical specification

Practice-based staff may wish to maintain autonomy within their work, but there is a tendency for large and remotely funded organisations, such as health care systems, to exercise quite stringent controls over minute details of operations. This may be exercised by hierarchically-placed managers, who are constrained themselves by conditions passed down from political sources in publicly funded health services (as through health service commissioners in the UK, for example) or from privately operated insurance companies in some other countries.

In Cowley's (1995b) analysis of the organisational arrangements in a community nursing unit, for example, communication was severely inhibited by extensive disjuncture and hierarchical separation between the different levels of staff. Three distinct and separate groups were apparent: practitioners, managers within the provider unit, and commissioners. A single loop of communication pertained, in which information was directed from the practice level through the managers to the purchasers. Controlling decisions about levels of funding, permitted types of practice and goals by which the work would be measured were directed from the commissioners back through the managers to the practitioners. The practitioners demonstrated no awareness of the deep and compassionate concern expressed by their senior managers for the difficulties encountered by both the overworked staff and the public they served, nor that the managers wished to involve them more in the decision-making processes. In turn, the commissioners demonstrated little understanding or interest in the complexities of clinical decision-making or the potential impact of their decisions on the point of service delivery.

There is a tendency for such fragmented and mechanistic organisations to develop a proliferation of rules, policies and procedures that may serve to restrict or obstruct self-organisation and learning within the system (Morgan and Ramirez 1983). The principle of minimum critical specification suggests that very few ground rules or enabling conditions are necessary within the organisation. This process involves choosing to place limits of action rather than forcing a choice of specific action, as required in mechanical design. This builds flexibility into the system as it allows a continuous redefining of goals and innovation in developing new actions according to what is happening in the environment and practice context.

The principle assumes the existence of reflection on the assumptions that guide action in the practice situation as well as external developments that have the potential to affect practice. Control within the practice setting is needed to act on those reflections, which illustrates the idea of 'double-loop learning' (Argyris & Schön 1978). In the community nursing setting outlined above, for example, double-loop learning would have involved information as well as control being directed from the commissioners to the practitioners, so they had a wider grasp of the difficulties pertaining at a strategic level. Keeping practice guidelines to the absolute minimum would make it possible for the nurses to have a high degree of autonomy at the practice level and to use the feed-back loop to exert control over the nature and format of those specifications.

This kind of organisational model assumes that all levels of workers are equally responsible for achieving the aims of the whole organisation, so there would be no reason to suppose that such autonomy would be exercised irresponsibly. A further assumption is that minimum regulation encourages reflective questioning and rational inquiry, rather than the mindless following of procedures and checklists so beloved of bureaucratic management systems, including, it must be said, the very ritually orientated and militaristic hierarchies that have long pervaded nursing organisations. Double-loop learning is an essential characteristic of a system that is able to learn from its own operations and to demonstrate the capacity for 'substantial rationality'. This is the third and last of the three holographic principles.

Substantial rationality

Professionalists tend to assume that the best and most effective way of assuring high quality care is through the maintenance of high professional standards, regulated by the profession itself and assessed through the unique experience of a single recipient of care. Their special claim to serve the public good rests on the supposed altruism embedded within their practice, which is guided by an ethically sound code of conduct; the UKCC provides such guidance for the nursing professions (UKCC 1992).

Managerialists working in the so-called 'not-for profit' sector might, quite reasonably, resent any suggestion that their labours are directed anywhere other than in the interests of the public their organisation serves. From this perspective, improved service to the public is obtained by good organisational management which ensures that everyone receives a high standard of care, evidenced by quality assurance across the organisation and in general terms. A professionalising intent is, perhaps, discernible within health care management, and many equivalent features, such as segmentation into different specialisms and an interest in ensuring that decisions are ethically sound, are beginning to emerge.

The idea of guidance on conduct is increasingly important in public life, and members of NHS boards are given clear guidance regarding expectations of their conduct, judgements and propriety (DoH 1994). There are numerous texts that provide guidance about the ethical principles required to underpin health care decisions (e.g., Seedhouse 1988, Wall 1989). Particular issues recur, such as economic decisions and rationing of services, perhaps beginning to indicate an emerging area of specialist knowledge. Despite this 'outside guidance', organisations such as the Institute of Health Service Management (IHSM) have developed a statement of primary values to guide their members in making decisions individually and within their organisation (IHSM 1997), representing a code of conduct developed internally by managers themselves. Whether or not managers are ever to be afforded 'professional status', or whether they would wish to seek it, may be a subject of great interest to sociologists. The interesting point to note for this chapter and this book is the extent to which there are increasingly shared agendas between professionals and managers.

A deep understanding of the ethical basis of practical action is required for an organisational system that demonstrates 'substantial rationality'. This is defined as the capacity for intelligent action based on a reflective understanding of the nature of the system and its context (Morgan and Ramirez 1983). Encouraging the use of intelligence and initiative among its members is intended to help make the organisation more substantially rational and effective in the longer term, even at the expense of short-term functional rationality. It requires the ability to challenge values, norms, policies and underlying assumptions that may cause difficulties, rather than simply aiming to solve problems that present themselves.

Questions, not answers

Taking a pragmatic stance, Marsick (1987) points out that there are limits to who can learn best under these 'holographic principles' and to the conditions within an organisation that facilitate or impede development. Organisations necessarily have some kind of instrumental focus associated with their primary purpose, whether that is to make a profit or provide health care. Not all individuals are equally ready to participate in decision-making and self-directed learning; nor is it possible for organisations to always change conditions such as hierarchy and centralised decision-making. Also, this is but one example of a 'worked through' model of organisational management; such examples abound and appear on the bookshelves daily. It is, nevertheless, a useful example for the purposes of this chapter and from which to introduce this text. Later chapters will outline other approaches and explain the major movements in preferred management and organisational styles.

At the start of this chapter, two options were offered: nursing might continue its quest for professional status or choose instead to define itself from a managerial focus. By this point, it is apparent that the traditional archetypes in either of those options do not have much to offer. However, the aspirations represented in managerialism and professionalism are changing; new visions are being set out for both spheres that, increasingly, follow a shared agenda and similar values. There is an enormously exciting potential for nursing and the population this group serves, if it is only possible to harness and capitalise on that momentum.

Sadly, the old ways are seriously entrenched and positive change is discussed far more often than it is achieved; in too many instances 'change fatigue' has led to inertia rather than the dynamism needed to motivate and excite innovation. There are enormous barriers to be overcome; the sheer complexity and interrelatedness of the systems in which nurses work can seem so daunting that achieving even small changes within known parameters can overwhelm. Nursing lacks status or power, and is often low on the list of health service priorities.

This book aims to help overcome that occasional sense of confusion and powerlessness by identifying some of the most influential aspects of these interrelated systems, holding them up to critical scrutiny and unravelling some of the taken-for-granted assumptions embedded within them. This opening chapter offers no clear conclusions, only insights that are picked up in the commentaries later in the text. Readers are invited to use these points as they read the rest of the text, to develop their own ideas and contribute collective thinking about nursing as an occupation and the nature of its particular contribution to human well-being. Hopefully some dialogue and debate will result. Positive action will only happen later, if enough nurses agree about the most suitable way to achieve forward progress in their occupation.

References

Argyris, C. & Schön, D. (1978) *Organisational Learning: a theory of action perspective.* Addison Wesley, Reading, Massachusetts.

Black, S. & Hagel, D. (1996) Developing an integrated nursing team approach. *Health Visitor,* **69** (7), 280–83.

Cohen, P. (1998) Breaking down the barriers: the new primary care act pilots. *Community Practitioner,* **71** (3), 93–4.

Cowley, S. (1995a) Health-as-process: a health visiting perspective. *Journal of Advanced Nursing,* 22, 433–41.

Cowley (1995b) Professional development and change in a learning organization. *Journal of Advanced Nursing,* 21, 965–74.

Daniels, A.K. (1987) Invisible work. *Social Problems,* **34** (5), 403–13.

Davies, C. (1995) *Gender and the Professional Predicament of Nursing.* Open University Press, Buckingham.

Davies, C. (1996a) Cloaked in a tattered illusion. *Nursing Times,* **92** (43), 44–6.

Davies, C. (1996b) A new vision of professionalism. *Nursing Times,* **92** (46), 54–6.

DoH (Department of Health) (1994) *Code of Conduct for NHS Boards.* HMSO, London.

Friedson, E. (1970) *Profession of Medicine: a study of applied knowledge.* Dodd, Mead and Co, New York.

Griffiths, P. & Evans, A. (1995) *Evaluation of a Nursing-led In-patient Service: an interim report.* King's Fund, London.

Hector, W. (1973) *The Work of Mrs Bedford Fenwick and the Rise of Professional Nursing.* Royal College of Nursing, London.

Humphreys, J. (1996) Educational commissioning by consortia: some theoretical and practical issues relating to qualitative aspects of British nurse education. *Journal of Advanced Nursing,* 24, 1288–99.

Hutchison, G., Addington-Hall, Bower, M., Austen, M. & Coombes, C. (1991) An evaluation of patient satisfaction with care provided by a multi-disciplinary cancer team. *European Journal of Cancer Care,* **1** (1), 15–18.

IHSM (1997) *Professional Code of Conduct and Statement of Values.* Institute of Health Service Management, London.

Iles, V. (1997) *Really Managing Health Care.* Open University Press, Buckingham.

Illich, I. (1976) The epidemics of modern medicine. Excerpts reproduced in *Health and Disease: a Reader* (1995) 2nd edn (eds B. Davey, A. Gray & C. Seale) pp. 237–42. Open University Press, Buckingham.

Jordan, S. (1994) Nurse practitioners: learning from the USA experience. *Health and Social Care in the Community*, 2, 173–86.

Kitson, A. (1987) A comparative analysis of lay-caring and professional (nursing) caring relationships. *International Journal of Nursing Studies*, **24** (2), 155–65.

Knowles, M. (1990) *The Adult Learner: a Neglected Species*, 4th edn. Gulf Publishing, Houston, Texas.

Kramer, M. (1974) *Reality Shock: why nurses leave nursing*. C.V. Mosby, St Louis.

Malin, N. & Teasdale, K. (1991) Caring versus empowerment: considerations for nursing practice. *Journal of Advanced Nursing*, 16, 657–62.

Marsick, V. (1987) *Learning in the Workplace*. Croom Helm, London.

Melia, K. (1984) Student nurses' construction of occupational socialisation. *Sociology of Health and Illness*, **6** (2), 132–51.

Melia, K. (1987) *Learning and Working: The occupational socialisation of nurses*. Tavistock, London.

Millerson, G. (1964) *The Qualifying Association*. Routledge, Kegan, Paul, London.

Mitchell, L. & Coats, M. (1997) The functional map of health and social care. In: *Interprofessional Working for Health and Social Care* (eds J. Ovretveit, P. Mathias, T. Thompson), pp. 157–87. Macmillan Press, Basingstoke.

Moline, J. (1986) Professionals and professions: a philosophical examination of an ideal. *Social Science and Medicine*, **22** (5), 501–508.

Morgan, G. & Ramirez, R. (1983) Action learning: a holographic metaphor to guide social change. *Human Relations*, 37, 1–28.

Morse, J., Bottorff, J., Neader, W. & Solberg, S. (1994) Comparative analysis of conceptualizations and theories of caring. In: *Contemporary Leadership Behaviour: Selected Readings* (eds E. Hein & M.J. Nicholson) 4th edn., pp. 25–42. J.B. Lippincott Company, Philadelphia.

Nyberg, J. (1994) The nurse as professnocrat. In: *Contemporary Leadership Behaviour: Selected Readings* (eds E. Hein & M.J. Nicholson) 4th edn, pp. 371–6. J.B. Lippincott Company, Philadelphia.

Onyett, S., Standen, R. & Peck, E. (1997) The challenge of managing community mental health teams. *Health and Social Care in the Community*, 5, 40–47.

Peters, T. & Waterman, R. (1982) *In Search of Excellence*. Warner Books, New York.

Porter, S. (1992) The poverty of professionalization: a critical analysis of strategies for the occupational advancement of nursing. *Journal of Advanced Nursing*, 17, 720–26.

Poulton, B. (1994) Primary health care team effectiveness: developing a constituency approach. *Health and Social Care in the Community*, 2, 77–84.

Rijke, R. (1993) Health in medical science; from determinism towards autonomy. In *Towards a New Science of Health* (eds R. Lafaille and S. Fulder) pp. 74–83. Routledge, London.

Robinson, J. (1991) Working with doctors: educational conditioning. *Nursing Times*, **6** (87) 28–31.

Schön, D. (1971) *Beyond the Stable State*. Temple Smith, London.

Schön, D. (1983) *The Reflective Practitioner: how professionals think in action*. Basic Books, New York.

Seedhouse, D. (1988) *Ethics: The Heart of Healthcare*. John Wiley and Sons, Chichester.

Smith, P. (1991) The nursing process: raising the profile of emotional care in nurse training. *Journal of Advanced Nursing*, 16, 74–81.

UKCC (1992) (3rd edn) *Code of Professional Conduct for the Nurse, Midwife and Health Visitor*. United Kingdom Central Council, London.

Wall, A. (1989) *Ethics and the Health Services Manager*. King's Fund, London.

Section 2
Nursing: The Ideal

Commentary: A Profession Based on Caring

The two chapters in this section reflect the archetypal view of nursing as a profession based on the central ideal of caring. Other social welfare professions make this claim too (Hugman 1991), but nursing's claim to labour around aspects of daily living means that it is widely assumed to be the ultimate caring profession by many professional nurses and by the general public.

Morrison and Cowley set the scene in Chapter 2, offering a basic celebration of nursing as caring in practice. Their chapter attempts to convey the passion and commitment felt by some nurses to this concept, and to explain why this amorphous ideal is considered so widely to be an essential basis on which to build the profession. Caring is presented as central, not for the good of nurses but because it is considered an essential component of a positive experience for patients. Although this chapter recognises the part played by other occupations, an attempt is made to convey caring by nurses as a distinctive part of their knowledge and skill; the growing research base to demonstrate how caring contributes to patient well-being is used to support the claim. That it is essentially 'for the public good' is considered almost axiomatic. However, there is a warning that the current recruitment crisis may be exacerbated if nurses are not allowed to exercise their 'caring' professionalism; this is a tacit recognition that nurses are not always afforded autonomy in practice to carry out this aspect of their work. Thus, from the start, the traditional model of professionalism becomes problematic, since the central ideal is not upheld.

Bergen takes a more sceptical and critical stance towards caring in Chapter 3; she clearly reveals interests and teaching drawn from a range of other professions, philosophy and research to refute any claims to exclusive knowledge and skills in this field. Even so, she demonstrates how nursing is particularly able to take this eclectic and contested concept and develop its theoretical, therapeutic, relational and ethical dimensions through the practice of caring for and about patients in changing situations. The archetypal aspects of traditional professionalism are not raised to any level of importance in this chapter. However, a convincing case is made to show how caring in modern nursing practice can enable interdependent decision-making, collective responsibility and patient involvement – all aspects of Davies' (1996) proposed 'new vision' of professionalism.

Together, the two chapters in this section show that nursing without caring would be unacceptable; its importance needs to be better acknowledged within health care systems. Other skills and knowledge are important in nursing as well, but implementing them within a caring framework is considered essential and provides the basis from which nursing lays traditional and modern claims to professionalism.

References

Davies, C. (1996) A new vision of professionalism. *Nursing Times*, **92** (46), 54–6.
Hugman, R. (1991) *Power in Caring Professions*. Macmillan, Basingstoke.

2 Idealised Caring: The Heart of Nursing

Kate Morrison and *Sarah Cowley*

Introduction

This chapter aims to explain why many nurses feel so strongly that caring lies at the very heart of nursing. The concept of caring is analysed from within the construct of nursing. The critique by Bergen (Chapter 3) will set the concept in the wider context of health and human care, in anticipation of the changes discussed in subsequent chapters. The chapter starts with a description of the special nature of nursing, outlined in Box 2.1.

Box 2.1: Caring in nursing.

John had never contemplated being ill. When he found an ulcerated lesion, he did not go to the doctor because he did not want to bother him. When at last he did go, the malignant, fungating lesion was beyond surgical help. During his last weeks at home he was weak and confined to bed. Betty, his wife, cared for him. She loved him very much, and at first declined professional nursing help because she wanted to do all the caring herself. But soon the lesion began to smell, and John became so thin that areas of pressure on his back started to break down.

When the community nurse, Sue, first arrived, she recognised John and Betty were two elderly and proud people whose values and beliefs had been shaped by the culture of living all their lives in a small Scottish village. As her relationship with them developed, Sue recognised the importance to John of having always been 'the man of the house'. When the three were together she allowed John to tease her about her driving, and they would all chat about changes in the village. When Sue and John were alone, she drew on her knowledge of wound care to relieve the odour and discomfort of the lesion. John felt a sense of spiritual as well as physical relief. He was not able to accept the terrible decay or raise the subject in conversation with Betty. Although married for 49 years, Betty and John needed Sue to act as mediator because of this illness that had come to separate them. Sue and John spent time together talking, she allowing him to tell in his own phrases, of the fears he had of dying, fears he would not worry his family with. She allowed the child inside the 75 year old patriarch to come through. Following Sue's visits John and Betty always felt soothed, and looked forward to the next visit. 'Aye, she's a rare lass,' he always said.

The night the lesion eroded a main artery and John began to bleed profusely, Betty rang Sue at home. She came straight away. She coped with the blood and the horror. Her presence calmed them. The doctor came, but there was nothing he could do. When it was all over, she and Betty washed John's body together.

This case study draws on the experiences of John and Betty, my father and mother-in-law. Their story relates a 'caring in nursing' event in which, from their perspective, the nurse demonstrated love, respect for others, commitment and compassion. She recognised the humanity in others and the need for their relationships to be fluid and adapting; she was never hurried, and listened and perceived Betty's needs as well as John's. Sue's technical skills were used to good effect and were underpinned by her commitment to maintain the quality of John's life during his last few weeks; this was clear to John and Betty and was appreciated by them. Betty felt that Sue gave her courage which helped her prepare for and bear her loss. The story encompasses many of the special attributes involved in nursing; it outlines the delivery of a high quality service that was perceived as caring.

Historically, caring has been considered synonymous with nursing (McFarlane 1976); more recently it is claimed as a substantive element and the essence of nursing (Leininger 1988a). However, caring involves skills which, in isolation, can be claimed by many occupations. Furthermore, new approaches to care organisation contingent on value for money reviews mean that personal care work, once the domain of nursing, is now (and possibly always has been) carried out increasingly by care assistants, with varying degrees of nursing supervision. The challenge for professional nursing, therefore, is to articulate more clearly what is meant by the concept of 'caring'. Professional nursing needs to justify claims to be paramount among the caring professions, and why this aspect of service provision should be allowed to make a claim on the public purse.

What is caring?

The term 'caring' originates from the Old English verb, *carian*, meaning 'to trouble oneself' (Dunlop 1986). This interpretation is still in common use along with dictionary definitions such as 'to have regard for', 'to provide physical needs and comfort', and 'to pay serious attention' (McLeod 1986). Nurses and nursing theorists have adopted a variety of ways of unravelling the nature of caring in nursing in order to examine and research it in further detail.

Dichotomy and science

Much of the literature highlights the dichotomy between emotional labour and technological skills of nurses to meet the varying needs of the one being cared for. Wild (1989), for example, separates the notions of 'caring for' and 'caring about'. In the former, the nurses' activities are predominantly physical interventions to compensate for the inability of the recipient to function independently; this includes elements of control, protection and taking over responsibility. Malin and Teasdale (1991) criticise the power imbalance inherent in the assumption that nurses have the right to take such decisions out of patients' hands.

Wild (1989) warns against the potential for 'caring for' activities to become routinised and robotic; she suggests conscious awareness of the need to 'care about' as a safeguard. This aspect of care is more concerned with affective aspects such as interest in and concern for; appropriate timing in re-instituting independence is the major corrective against the dehumanising tendency in routinised care provision. In a philosophical analysis of caring, Griffin (1983) also describes the importance of the nurse recognising patients' physical and emotional needs. Tronto (1989) claims that this is dependent on the carer having particular knowledge of the one cared for, and a profound self-knowledge, so that his or her self needs are not unconsciously projected onto the one being cared for.

This dichotomous approach of separating out physical and emotional aspects to care appears especially prevalent when nurses specialise in technical health fields, formerly the realm of doctors, and where a biomedical model is the norm. Colliere (1986) claims that nurses who move into technical fields do so because they wish to fit in with the 'so-called scientific rationale', thereby evading the interpersonal aspects of nursing caring. Alternatively it could be said that nurses who push out the boundaries of their clinical practice are applying the art of caring to new spheres of patient care.

Dunlop (1986) also draws attention to the dualism implicit in notions of curing and caring, along with the associated connotations of gender and social class. She questions whether a science of caring is possible, but dichotomous assumptions about caring make the possibility of research more feasible, since some aspects can be separated out and measured to assess impact and effectiveness.

Holism and humanism

In contrast to this dualistic approach, Watson (1985) advocates that caring in nursing concerns itself with the uniqueness of the individual, giving priority to the total person in their social context, rather than to their organic pathogens or health disorders. This theory draws heavily on the phenomenological-existentialist view that the person being cared for will perceive a relief from existential loneliness, feel safe and understood (Watson 1985), which is valuable to both carer and those cared for. This is a core aspect of all reciprocally caring relationships and is not unique to nursing.

A holistic approach involves the joint application of scientific knowledge and interpersonal skills identified as separate aspects of caring in the dichotomised descriptions outlined above. Benner (1984) refers to these two parts of caring as the instrumental and expressive aspects of nursing. She warns against considering caring as an art only, as that would risk ignoring caring as a subject of scholarly enquiry. Leininger also embraces both emotional and physical aspects in her interpretation of caring in nursing, explaining that:

'Professional caring embodies the cognitive and deliberate goals, processes and acts of professional persons ... providing assistance to others, and expressing attitudes and actions of concern for them...'

(Leininger 1988b: 46).

Leininger and Watson have both developed significant theories of caring in nursing using different approaches; they each stress the need for a science of nursing caring. Leininger (1988b) places an emphasis on the transcultural context of care in relation to human growth, knowledge and practice, while Watson (1985) concentrates on the importance of transpersonal relationships and the existentialist view of human worth. Koldjeski (1990) developed a model to integrate the major perspectives proposed by Leininger and Watson; she achieved this by identifying the humanistic 'essences' and scientific 'entities' embedded in the concept of caring.

In his classic work on human caring, Mayeroff (1971) suggests all caring relationships exhibit a common pattern; he elicited the concepts of devotion, knowledge, alternating rhythms, patience, honesty, trust, humility, hope and courage. The outcome of a combined study of patients and nurses by Wolf *et al.* (1994) revealed five dimensions of the process of nurse-caring: 'respectful deference to other', 'assurance of human presence', 'positive connectedness', 'professional knowledge and skill', and 'attentive to other's experience' (Wolf *et al.* 1994, p. 110).

The nurse needs the psychological ability to care and an intrinsic desire to promote goal-directed, interpersonal relationships with patients, which make use of implicit nursing knowledge and skills. Caring is possible in any nursing interaction if the environment allows this; for example, it would not be possible to care holistically for critically ill patients without appropriate equipment or if staff–patient ratios were too low. Not only would this be a threat to patient safety, but, '... the creation of an expectation to care without the provision to fulfil that expectation leads to despair and disillusionment'. (Radsma 1994, p. 447)

Theorists such as Noddings (1984) claim that caring cannot take place without reciprocity and equity, and there is a wealth of research into health care relationships to demonstrate the relevance of this (e.g., Thorne & Robinson 1988, Chalmers 1992). However, caring in nursing does not demand this of every encounter. Nursing an unconscious patient involves equity of both parties as human beings, but will not lead to a reciprocal relationship. Relating in a reciprocal way to forensic patients in secure mental hospitals or aggressive attenders at an accident and emergency unit might be downright dangerous to all concerned; but ensuring a person's nursing needs are met despite unsociable behaviour is an expression of human caring.

Caring as a metaphor

Some of the most passionate and extravagant language is used by commentators who seek to justify nursing by using caring as a metaphor. It is variously described as, '... the candle that lights the dark' (Benner & Wrubel 1988, p. 1073) and as the common thread that runs through nursing: 'like the string in a necklace, it holds all the beads together' (Duke & Copp 1992, p. 40). Gaut (1993) suggests it is parallel to love, a euphemism also used by Jacono (1993) who proposes that nursing's fascination with defining the concept is powered by an innate fear of caring.

It is claimed that the capacity to care is inherent in human nature (Carper 1979, Brown *et al.* 1992), and is 'a deep inchoate quest which does not have definable objects' (van Hooft 1996, p. 84). For Bottorff (1991) concepts of caring should be elaborated and combined so that caring in nursing can be distinguished from other forms of caring. Bottorff's vision suggests a need for symmetry and fusion of these foci that will transform nursing caring into a 'holophrase'.

It may be argued that the extreme is necessary to help us see the obvious, to uncover 'the significance in the taken-for-granted' as in phenomen-ological research (van Manen 1990, p. 8). However, such unconventional and intense terminology is not universally acceptable and it may be simply off-putting. Barker *et al.* (1995), for example, complain that Watson's theory is couched in such obfuscatory, 'new age' language that the concept of caring becomes a one-sided, emotional self-indulgence which has no place in human interaction and the helping relationship. Opponents of multi-dimensional or simple definitions defend the mystery inherent in concepts such as love and caring (Marcel 1956). To reduce caring to an entity or taxonomy of actions spelled out in universal rules may be considered philosophically naive (Phillips 1993, Dunlop 1986), and Kitson (1996) suggests that finding new metaphors and images that communicate the essence of nursing will be a hard task. Nevertheless, Barker *et al.* (1995) warn against allowing the quest of defining caring to become 'the raison d'etre of nursing'.

Gender and the caring imperative

Traditionally, nursing has been a predominantly female profession and most of its virtuous caring qualities such as, 'concern for the welfare of others, nurturant traits ... interpersonal sensitivity, emotional expressive-ness and a gentle personal style' (Friedman 1987, p. 65) are strongly associated with society's ideal of femininity. The lay notion of nurse as 'angel', although slowly changing, has been stubbornly coloured by the ascendancy of nursing's history and influence of gender. Care of the sick and dying was considered, throughout history, to be the works of duty, charity and mercy. In many parts of the world, nursing became formalised under religious orders, and in the nineteenth century it was viewed as a vocation only for pious women (Nelson 1995) whose '... moral obligation to obedience and service was passed on to generations of nurses' (Radsma 1994, p. 446). When nurse training began, Colliere (1986) suggests the expressive aspects of caring were a legacy from nursing nuns who practised dedication and devotion. The instrumental aspects of nursing were developed in association with doctors and are often interpreted as skills lent by male doctors, to whom the female nurse was in service.

Rafael (1996) refers to the pervasive androcentric values of Western society whose 'male-stream' ethics of beneficence and rights-based justice have capitalised on women's ability to care both in the private and public domain. As a female workforce, nursing has experienced twofold the exploitation of femininity as, '. . . in a traditional view . . . caring in nursing practice . . . is not recognised as requiring any particular knowledge or skill; it simply comes "naturally" to women' (Rafael 1996, p. 8).

Davies (1995) also links this professional predicament in nursing to gender, with staff transience and workload being the main vehicles used to undermine the value that nurses might, themselves, place on the work they do. Managers who, 'limit caring time and require concrete, measurable outcomes to justify caring actions' (Morse *et al.* 1990, p. 12) lower morale in nurses, ultimately leading to burnout. In the absence of management recognition, Benner and Wrubel (1989, p. 373) recommend social support from other nurses subjected to similar stresses as the 'most effective way to reduce burnout and distress'.

The whole idea of caring has, perhaps, been trivialised by media use in promoting consumer products such as household detergents. It has also become a symbolic word in diverse health areas, including logo designs for NHS trusts and provision of complementary medicine. Rawnsley (1990) argues that this highlights the importance of nurses articulating ways in which caring and nursing are uniquely integral. Difficulties arise in that a viable ideology is needed that will, 'help them [nurses] adjust to the continual demands of patients and an ever more bureaucratised, cost conscious and rationalised work setting' (Reverby 1987, p. 9). Advancing the value of caring to 'decision makers familiar with evaluating alternatives based on quantified variables' is not easy (Valentine 1989, p. 29).

Summary: caring in nursing

Caring in nursing may be described in dichotomous ways: associated with scientific and technical skills, or viewed as a holistic, central part of all nursing, which is a mainly humanistic approach. Working to the first description is acknowledged as problematic for patients because of the tendency to promote mechanistic 'production-line' approaches to care, but it is, apparently, quite widely supported within organisations because it is potentially economical. The second view may be reviled because of its association with extravagant terminology and overt feminism in defence of nursing work, but arguably the concepts enshrined within this concept of caring remain central to the quality of nursing provision.

A compilation of these attributes of caring is shown in Fig. 2.1; this is drawn from the works of Mayeroff (1971), Griffin (1983), Benner (1984), Noddings (1984), Watson (1985), Leininger (1988b), Hall (1989), Tronto (1989), Valentine (1989), Koldjeski (1990), Marck (1990), Morse *et al.* (1990), Holden (1991), Brown *et al.* (1992), Boykin and Schoenhofer (1993). The

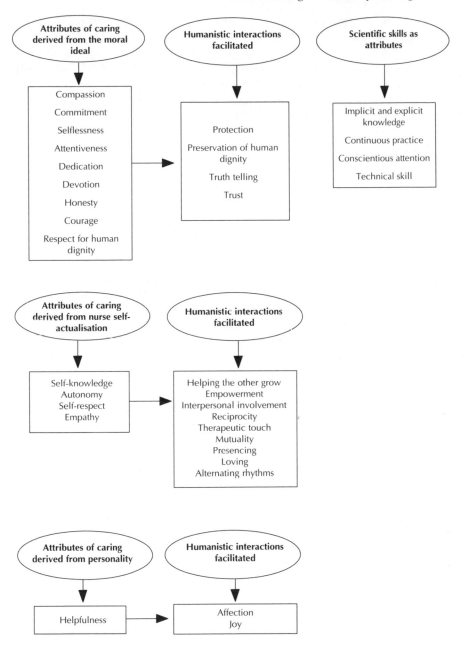

Fig. 2.1 Care theorists' attributes of caring in nursing.

nurse–patient interactions facilitated by these attributes are shown in the second column. The scientific, instrumental attributes of caring in nursing are listed in the third column, to demonstrate that, although part of the whole, their contribution, according to care theorists, is less than that of moral ideal and self-actualisation attributes.

A review of definitions shows a predilection for describing caring in nursing as an interpersonal skill (Watson 1988, Gendron 1990, Cohen 1991, Shiber and Larson 1991, Condon 1992, Jaggar 1995, Webb 1996) and humanistic interaction (Leininger 1988b, Forrest 1989, Chipman 1991) which protects and enhances the human dignity of others (Fry 1989) helping them to grow and self actualise (Gaut 1993) by showing concern, regard and consideration (Carper 1979, Graham 1983). Caring is seen as a moral ideal (Condon 1992), which is the foundation for an ethic of caring (Noddings 1984).

Why caring?

If caring was only about the professionalising self-interest of nurses, it could not be sustained. It can only be justified if there is a benefit to be gained by those on the receiving end of care. Morse *et al.* (1991) suggest that the moral attributes of caring in nursing result in ethical nursing behaviour at the personal and professional level, whereas the nurse's therapeutic interventions result in a change in the patient's condition on the basis of nursing competency.

Hall (1989) considers the interpersonal encounter of caring involves the beliefs and philosophies of those concerned, individual goals, practices and acts – the minimum of which may just be physical presence – and emotions and feelings that may be extreme. He defines the objective of caring as protection, prevention, help and support and asks what it is that makes people want to care when there is no pre-existing emotional or social attachment? Noddings (1984) suggests that the capacity to care for those outside the family circle is eternalised by humans' memories of being cared for, and Griffin (1983) states that the prolonged and reliable attention people pay to their children and relatives is of central relevance to nursing.

Benefits for patients

The outcomes of caring are difficult to quantify through research because of the ethical contraindications of using control groups and they may have multiple causes which 'can rarely be directly linked with specific causes of care' (Shiber & Larson 1991, p. 64). However, some surveys have been undertaken and there is qualitative research that helps to shed light on how patients perceive and experience care.

In a phenomenological study of male and female patients' interpretations of nurse caring, Riemen (1986) found that both groups rated highly reassurance, a gentle approach and valuing of the individual. Larson's (1984) quantitative study of cancer patients' perceptions of caring found that patients prioritised the attributes of nurse accessibility, monitoring and following through, suggesting a patient need for reassurance through nurse presence. Patients also chose technical competencies such as ability to give injections and manage technical equipment as indicators of caring nurse behaviours.

The patient's confidence in the nurse's ability to provide physical care and treatment was considered fundamental to the experience of care (Brown 1986). The importance of congruent perceptions of need was emphasised in this qualitative analysis of views from 50 acute medical and surgical patients. Likewise, Cronin and Harrison's (1988) research with cardiac patients reported nurses' knowledge of equipment and their overall competency to be most significant. These studies all support the view that caring has a practical and technical, as well as an affective and emotional, aspect.

Nurse personality traits were important to patients, who looked for cheerfulness (Mayer 1987). Patients felt that cold, impersonal facial expression, lack of eye contact and hurried pace excluded them from caring interactions with nurses (Drew 1986). These findings indicate that people's vulnerability in unfamiliar environments is often expressed through the primeval need for survival and safety, congruent with hierarchical theories of human need. Prior assumptions that nurses have inherent altruism and empathy could also influence the choice of safety factors coming high on patient agendas.

Halldorsdottir (1991) studied the experiences of patients who felt that they had been treated in an uncaring way by hospital nurses. At first the patients were puzzled by, and disbelieving of, the nurses' behaviours. They described feelings of betrayal and loss of identity. The patients' perceived vulnerability during a time of sickness and need was greatly increased and their memories of the uncaring encounters had a greater effect than any caring encounters, staying with them for a long time and negatively influencing their views of health care.

Nurses' perceptions

Nurses' perceptions of caring attributes show some divergence from those of patients. Nurses, as research subjects, give priority to the humanistic and cognitive aspects of caring. Dyson's (1996) study supported this philosophy in finding that ability to give of self, consideration, sensitivity, motivation and communication skills were highly valued by nurses. A survey of 1430 nurses in Scotland showed that listening to patients was seen as a caring attribute, whereas sharing of their own personal problems with the patient was an uncaring attribute (Watson & Lea 1997), succinctly illustrating the moral attribute of selflessness. Larson (1987) and von Essen and Sjödén (1991) all found that nurses considered listening, comforting and therapeutic touch to be specific indicators of caring in nursing.

No studies were found that expressed technical skills as being predominantly significant in the nurses' view. It could be that attributes of caring as described by the nurses in these studies indicate a transcendence from the craftsmanship of nursing, bringing a completeness to the concept. Salvage (1990) questions the recurrent priority nurses give to quasi-psychotherapeutic patient–nurse relationships, suggesting that patients' immediate concerns are likely to be relief from pain and discomfort. Patient concerns will vary depending on context. The therapeutic effect of a patient-nurse relationship is likely to be determined by the patient's wishes and the reason for, and length of, the encounter.

Student nurses in Chipman's (1991) study highlighted the fundamental aspects of meeting physical needs such as pain relief, but also included paying attention and fostering self-esteem. At the other end of the nursing spectrum, Komorita *et al.* (1991) interviewed 110 senior female nurses, the majority being nurse educators. From a given scale, the nurses identified as the three most important attributes: comforting through listening, enabling patient expression of fears and promoting autonomy.

Figure 2.2 is compiled from the attributes of nursing-caring put forward by patients and nurses in the published works of Larson (1984), Drew (1986), Larson (1986), Riemen (1986), Larson (1987), Mayer (1987), Cronin and Harrison (1988), Chipman (1991), von Essen and Sjödén (1991), Komorita *et al.* (1991), Morrison (1991), Wolf *et al.* (1994), Kyle (1995), Dyson (1996), Watson and Lea (1997). Although core attributes of the moral ideal and nurse self-actualisation are comparable to those in Fig. 2.1, there is greater emphasis on the attributes of caring derived from nurse personality and the scientific skills.

Nurses were more aware of the moral attributes than patients. Patients did not put forward ideas for attributes of caring derived from nurse self-actualisation, but recognised the ensuing products of motivation and empathy, in that they identified perception of needs and concerns, presencing and promotion of autonomy as significant attributes. A comparison of Figs 2.1 and 2.2 shows that nurses share the care theorists' criteria of moral attributes, a factor which could be the result of personal reflection and/or nurse education. Despite the weight given to technical skills in patients' perceived attributes compared to nurses, there is, overall, more congruence of perceived attributes of caring between patients and nurses in the clinical environment, than between nurses and care theorists.

Why caring in nursing?

In the concept of caring in nursing there will be shifts in meaning over time and fusion with related concepts such as altruism, empathy or love. Benner and Wrubel (1989) saw the concept of altruism not as a selfless response to another's need, but as a consequence of caring. In their view caring brings about a mutual realisation of human interdependence which fosters altruism. Synthesising caring with empathy provides a humanistic foundation for nursing care (Olsen 1991). Morse *et al.* (1992) prefer the term 'emotive engagement' to empathy, and propose it as the essence of the nurse–patient helping relationship.

Caring is seen by Fromm (1957) as a basic element of love, but he states that caring must be infused with knowledge or it becomes blind. Kitson (1996) speaks of the giving out and giving away of professional knowledge as being the heart of nursing. The argument is not whether these qualities exist in other helping professions such as social work or teaching, because

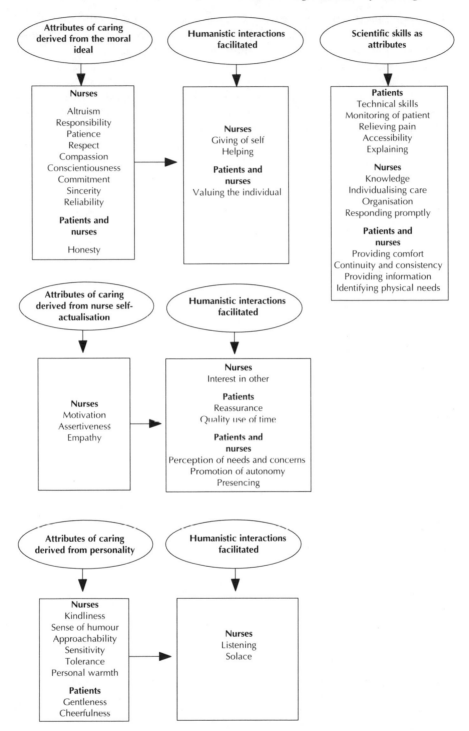

Fig. 2.2 Patients' and nurses' perceived attributes of caring.

of course they do. It is that caring is so strongly bound to 'the moral and social ideals of nursing' (Fry 1989) that, without it, nursing is diminished and void. Patients may only articulate their feelings about caring if they perceive it to be missing.

The benefit to human lives is implicit in caring. It is difficult to measure and for those who seek value for money, will not equate with hard evidence of clinical effectiveness. If the concept of caring in nursing becomes subsumed by an ideology of outcome measurements and 'techno-care', then cost-driven managers could weaken nursing by legitimising only the scientific nursing skills, which can then be classified and redistributed.

This may be counter-productive, partly because it would potentially decrease the job satisfaction for those motivated into nursing precisely because it offers an opportunity for expressing their caring ideals. The knock-on effect in terms of recruitment and retention is unpredictable, but may be greater than the expense of ensuring the service values the caring skills inherent in nursing. Furthermore, the experience of being a patient receiving a nursing provision that is devoid of caring would hardly accord with ideas of high quality service. Those who choose to practise as nurses need to acknowledge and articulate the worth of carrying out the practical and technical skills of nursing within a context of caring, for the benefit of those on the receiving end of this human care.

References

Barker, P.J., Reynolds, W. & Ward, T. (1995) The proper focus of nursing: a critique of the 'caring' ideology. *International Journal of Nursing Studies*, **32**(4), 386–97.

Benner, P. (1984) *From Novice to Expert*. Addison-Wesley, Menlo Park, California.

Benner, P., Wrubel J. (1988) Caring comes first. *American Journal of Nursing*. **88**(8), 1072–75.

Benner, P. & Wrubel, J. (1989) *The Primacy of Caring: Stress and Coping in Health and Illness*. Addison Wesley, Menlo Park.

Bottorff, J. (1991) Nursing: A practical science of caring. *Advances in Nursing Science*, **14**(1), 26–39.

Boykin, A. & Schoenhofer, S. (1993) *Nursing as Caring*. National League for Nursing Press, New York.

Brown, L. (1986) The experience of care: patient perspectives. *Topics in Clinical Nursing*, **8** (2) 56–62.

Brown, J., Kitson, A. & McKnight, T. (1992) *Challenges in Caring*. Chapman and Hall, London.

Carper, B. (1979) The ethics of caring. *Advances in Nursing Science*, **1**(3), 11–20.

Chalmers, K. (1992) Giving and receiving: an empirically derived theory on health visiting practice. *Journal of Advanced Nursing*, 17, 1317–25.

Chipman, Y. (1991) Caring: its meaning and place in the practice of nursing. *Journal of Nursing Education*, **30**(4), 171–5.

Cohen, J. (1991) Two portraits of caring: a comparison of the artists, Leininger and Watson. *Journal of Advanced Nursing*, 16, 899–909.

Colliere, M. (1986) Invisible care and invisible women as health care providers. *International Journal of Nursing Studies*, **23**(2), 95–112.

Condon, E. (1992) Nursing and the caring metaphor: gender and political influences on an ethics of care. *Nursing Outlook*, **40**(1), 14–19.

Cronin, S. & Harrison, B. (1988) Importance of nurse caring behaviours as perceived by patients after myocardial infarction. *Heart and Lung*, **17**(4), 374–80.

Davies, C. (1995) *Gender and the Professional Predicament of Nursing*. Open University Press, Buckingham.

Drew, N. (1986) Exclusion and confirmation: a phenomenology of patients' experiences with caregivers. *IMAGE Journal of Nursing Scholarship*, **18**(2), 39–43.

Duke, S. & Copp, G. (1992) Hidden nursing. *Nursing Times*, **88** (17), 40–42.

Dunlop, M. (1986) Is a science of caring possible? *Journal of Advanced Nursing*, 11, 661–70.

Dyson, J. (1996) Nurses' conceptualizations of caring attitudes and behaviours. *Journal of Advanced Nursing*, **23**(6), 1263–9.

Forrest, D. (1989) The experience of caring. *Journal of Advanced Nursing*, 14, 815–23.

Friedman, M. (1987) Beyond caring: the de-moralization of gender. In: *Justice and Care: Essential Readings in Feminist Ethics* (1995) (ed. V. Held) pp. 61–77. Westview, Colorado.

Fromm, E. (1957) *The Art of Loving*. Thorsons, London.

Fry, S. (1989) Towards a theory of nursing ethics. *Advances in Nursing Science*, **11**(4), 9–22.

Gaut, T. (1993) Caring: a vision of wholeness for nursing. *Journal of Holistic Nursing*, **11**(2), 164–71.

Gendron, D. (1990) Learning caring behaviour in an integrated manner. In: *The Caring Imperative in Education* (eds M. Leininger & J. Watson) pp. 277–84. National League for Nursing, New York.

Graham, H. (1983) Caring: A labour of love. In: *A Labour of Love* (eds J. Finch & D. Groves). Routledge, London.

Griffin, A. (1983) A philosophical analysis of caring in nursing. *Journal of Advanced Nursing*, 8, 289–95.

Hall, J. (1989) Towards a psychology of caring. *British Journal of Clinical Psychology*, 29, 129–44.

Halldorsdottir, S. (1991) Five basic modes of being with another. In: *Caring: The Compassionate Healer* (eds D.A. Gaut & M.M. Leininger) pp. 37–49. National League for Nursing Press, New York.

Holden, R. (1991) An analysis of caring, attributions, contributions and resolutions. *Journal of Advanced Nursing*, 16, 893–8.

Jacono, B. (1993) Caring is loving. *Journal of Advanced Nursing*, 18, 192–4.

Jaggar, A. (1995) Caring as a feminist practice of moral reason. In: *Justice and Care: Readings in Feminist Ethics* (ed. V. Held) pp. 179–201. Westview, Colorado.

Kitson, A.L. (1996) Does nursing have a future? *British Medical Journal*, **313** (7072), 1647–51.

Koldjeski, D. (1990) Toward a theory of professional nursing caring: a unifying perspective. In: *The Caring Imperative in Education* (eds M. Leininger & J. Watson) pp. 45–57. National League for Nursing, New York.

Komorita, N., Doehring, K. & Hirchet, P. (1991) Perceptions of caring by nurse educators. *Journal of Nursing Education*, **30**(1), 23–9.

Kyle, T. (1995) The concept of caring: a review of the literature. *Journal of Advanced Nursing*, 21, 506–14.

Larson, P. (1984) Important nurse caring behaviours perceived by patients with cancer. *Oncology Nursing Forum*, **11**(6), 46–50.

Larson, P. (1986) Cancer nurses' perceptions of caring. *Cancer Nursing*, **9**(2), 86–91.

Larson, P. (1987) Comparison of cancer patients' and professional nurses' perceptions of important nurse caring behaviours. *Heart and Lung*, **16**(2), 187–93.

Leininger, M. (1988a) Caring: a central focus of nursing and health care services. In: *Care: The Essence of Nursing and Health* (ed. M. Leininger), pp. 45–59. Wayne State University Press, Detroit.

Leininger, M. (1988b) Leininger's theory of nursing: cultural care diversity and universality. *Nursing Science Quarterly*, **1**(4), 152–60.

McFarlane, J. (1976) A charter for caring. *Journal of Advanced Nursing*, 1, 187–96.

Malin, N. & Teasdale, K. (1991) Caring versus empowerment: considerations for nursing practice. *Journal of Advanced Nursing*, 16, 657–62.

Marcel, G. (1956) *The Philosophy of Existentialism*. Citadel Press, New York.

Marck, P. (1990) Therapeutic reciprocity: a caring phenomenon. *Advances in Nursing Science*, **13**(1), 49–59.

Mayer, D. (1987) Oncology nurses' versus cancer patients' perceptions of nurse caring behaviours: a replication study. *Oncology Nursing Forum*, **14**(3), 48–52.

Mayeroff, M. (1971) *On Caring*. Harper and Row, New York.

McLeod, W. (ed) (1986) *The Collins Dictionary and Thesaurus*. Collins, London.

Morrison, P. (1991) The caring attitude in nursing practice: a repertory grid study of trained nurses' perceptions. *Nurse Education Today*, 11, 3–12.

Morse, J., Solberg, S., Neander, W., Bottorff, J. & Johnson, J. (1990) Concepts of caring and caring as a concept. *Advances in Nursing Science*, **13**(1), 1–14.

Morse, J., Bottorff, J., Neander, W. & Solberg, S. (1991) Comparative analysis of conceptualizations and theories of caring. *IMAGE Journal of Nursing Scholarship*, **23**(2), 119–26.

Morse, J., Bottorf, J., Anderson, G., O'Brien, B. & Solberg, S. (1992) Beyond empathy: expanding expressions of caring. *Journal of Advanced Nursing*, 17, 809–21.

Nelson, S. (1995) Humanism in nursing: the emergence of the light. *Nursing Inquiry*, **2**(1), 36–43.

Noddings, N. (1984) *Caring: A Feminist Approach to Ethics and Moral Education*. University of California Press, Berkeley, California.

Olsen, D. (1991) Empathy as an ethical and philosophical basis for nursing. *Advances in Nursing Science*, **14**(1), 62–75.

Phillips, P. (1993) A deconstruction of caring. *Journal of Advanced Nursing*, 18, 1554–58.

Radsma, J. (1994) Caring and nursing: a dilemma. *Journal of Advanced Nursing*, 20, 444–9.

Rafael, A. (1996) Power and caring: a dialectic in nursing. *Advances in Nursing Science*, **19** (1), 3–17.

Rawnsley, M. (1990) Of human bonding: the context of nursing as caring. *Advances in Nursing Science*, **13** (1), 41–8.

Reverby, S. (1987) *Ordered to Care*. Cambridge University Press, Cambridge.

Riemen, D. (1986) The essential structure of a caring interaction: doing phenomenology. In: *Nursing Research: A Qualitative Perspective* (eds P. Munhall & C. Oiler) pp. 85–108.

Salvage J. (1990) The theory and practice of the 'new nursing'. *Nursing Times*, **86**(4), 42–5.

Shiber, S. & Larson, E. (1991) Evaluating the quality of caring: structure, process and outcome. *Holistic Nursing Practice*, **5**(3), 57–66.

Thorne, S. & Robinson, C. (1988) Reciprocal trust in health care relationships. *Journal of Advanced Nursing*, 13, 782–9.

Tronto, J. (1989) Women and caring: what can feminists learn about morality from caring? In: *Justice and Care: Essential Readings in Feminist Ethics* (1995) (ed. V. Held) pp. 101–15. Westview, Colorado.

Valentine, K. (1989) Caring is more than kindness: modelling its complexities. *Journal of Nursing Administration*, **19**(11), 28–34.

van Hooft, S. (1996) Bioethics and caring. *Journal of Medical Ethics*, **22**(2), 83–89.

van Manen, M. (1990) *Researching Lived Experience*. Althouse, Ontario.

von Essen, L. & Sjödén, P. (1991) Patient and staff perceptions of caring: review and replication. *Journal of Advanced Nursing*, 16, 1363–74.

Watson, J. (1985) *Nursing: The Philosophy and Science of Caring*. University Press of Colorado, Colorado.

Watson, J. (1988) *Nursing: Human Science and Human Care. A Theory of Nursing*, National League for Nursing, New York.

Watson, R. & Lea, A. (1997) The caring dimensions inventory (CDI): content validity, reliability and scaling. *Journal of Advanced Nursing*, 25, 87–94.

Webb, C. (1996) Caring, curing, coping: towards an integrated model. *Journal of Advanced Nursing*, **23**(5), 960–68.

Wild, D. (1989) Caring for and caring about the elderly – defining the dynamics. *Senior Nurse*, **9**(6), 22–24.

Wolf, Z., Giardino, E., Osborne, P. & Ambrose, M. (1994) Dimensions of nurse caring. *IMAGE Journal of Nursing Scholarship*, **26**(2), 107–11.

3   An Analysis of Caring

Ann Bergen

Most, if not all occupations are underpinned by some relatively enduring ideals which help construct the social identity of the occupation and make its work both possible and recognisable. There are a bewildering number of theories and models which purport to represent the essence of nursing, and there are few occupations whose members have given such attention to making these ideals explicit (Bradshaw 1995). I do not intend to rehearse theories and models of nursing here, but to focus instead on one ideal which has, above all others, become associated with nursing practice – that of 'caring'. This chapter pursues the analysis of caring in relation to nursing that was started in Chapter 2.

In the following sections various typologies of care, as presented in the literature, will be explored for their compatibility with identifiable values in nursing, so that any enduring conceptualisation of 'nursing care' may be uncovered. The challenge of establishing a framework which is sufficiently focused and of adequate breadth, will serve as a backdrop to the analyses of different aspects and contexts of nursing which follow in Section 3.

Perspectives on care and caring

Although few would disagree with the assertion of Clifford (1995) that caring is a concept fundamental to the human experience, there are difficulties inherent in supporting, and in extracting the meanings contained within, this axiom. There is little consensus in the literature in terms of definitions of care (Lea & Watson 1996, Webb 1996), and those definitions that do exist lack specificity (Clifford 1995). One of the main problems appears to be that caring is what Benner and Wrubel (1989) call 'culturally invisible'; they, along with Smith (1992), ascribe the difficulties of capturing the gestures of care to the fact that it has traditionally been seen as 'women's natural work', that is, intuitive and instinctive.

This is clearly inadequate, even as a quasi-explanation, not only to these writers but also to commentators such as Warelow (1996) who contend that a theory of feminist ethics itself is too constraining as an interpretive framework for care. It also gives rise to a number of questions, which have been articulated over recent years: can care go beyond the images outlined above (Smith 1992)? Is care observable in the care giver or only identified by the recipient (Savage 1995)? From whose perspective should definitions of care be taken if these differ (Clifford 1995)? Have appropriate methods been developed to research this (Savage 1995)?

This last question is probably the most fundamental. A given perspective on care will depend on the underlying orientation in terms of theory development, and this, in turn, will have implications for nursing relevance. Lea and Watson (1996) describe a quantitative–qualitative continuum of theories, ranging from that of Watson (1988), taking an extreme existentialist position which argues for a holistic, multi-perspective approach to care, through Leininger (1981) and Orem (1980) to Gaut (1983), who takes a reductionist view that caring can be broken down into behavioural tasks and thus analysed.

Stances which represent both ends of this continuum are not without support and criticism. Clifford (1995) argues that, without operational definitions and behavioural designations, the scientific study of caring is limited. However, Webb (1996) after listing 32 defining characteristics gleaned from the literature, concludes that work on care still largely ignores the care recipient's views, except in limited, patient-satisfaction type surveys. Webb does acknowledge that the advent of more sophisticated research methods, such as the Q Sort (for instance the 'CARE Q' of Larson (1984)) is an attempt to overcome the limitations of earlier structured questionnaires, in that they allow greater opportunity to express the respondent's 'vision of reality'. However, this technique, in turn, has been subjected to criticism by Lea and Watson (1996) because it imposes and assumes the dimensions of care which respondents are asked to rate, and because small sample sizes are generally used in what still amounts to a forced-choice method of eliciting data. Moreover, such studies do tend to indicate a disparity between care giver and recipient views.

On the other hand, these writers also comment that the more qualitative approaches to the research of care tend to emphasise the nature of the carer, rather than the tasks and processes of caring, and therefore bring their own disadvantages. To overcome the limitations of both positions, Lea and Watson (1996) perceive a need to adopt a way forward which will harness the strengths of ethnographic and phenomenological methods, in order to reduce the inventories of caring attitudes already identified to their underlying dimensions. At the same time, they say, this needs to be done in a way which will withstand scrutiny from the scientific community.

Components of care

Although this challenge laid down by Lea and Watson (1996) remains, Morse *et al.* (1992) have put forward a framework which breaks down the notion of care into different (though interrelated) component dimensions, and which, therefore, provides a useful basis for conceptual analysis. The first of these, caring as a human trait, basically reiterates Clifford's (1995) 'care as fundamental' approach and, therefore, will not be expanded on here. However, an adapted version of the remaining dimensions will be used to frame a further consideration of the literature.

Care as an affect and care as a therapeutic intervention

Care as affect (extending self and emotions into the caring situation) and care as therapeutic intervention (planned and given) are not necessarily seen as antithetical in Morse *et al.'s* (1992) framework, but a dualism of similar characteristics is detectable in much of the recent literature and so the two dimensions can be usefully considered together.

The often quoted distinction in the literature between 'caring about' and 'caring for' has been discussed in some depth by Savage (1995). The former ideal, which signifies an attachment or emotional relationship but implies little about caring as a practical activity, is opposed to the latter impression of providing for needs ('therapy') without any necessary affinity or affection. This is often associated with what Savage (1995) sees as a false dichotomy between informal and formal spheres of care, or what Smith (1992) has described as care in the private and public arenas. And, again, the feminist ethic has been adopted to inform this dualist debate; for Gilligan (1982) stereotypical views suggest a splitting of care that 'relegates' (her word) its expressive capacities to women, while placing the associated instrumental ability within the masculine domain.

At the heart of this debate there appears to be a difficulty in accommodating the acknowledged affective aspect of caring within the professional culture to which many 'people orientated' occupations currently aspire. Smith's (1992) seminal analysis of this issue, based on a critique of the work of Hochschild (1983), may be helpful as a basis from which to discuss where nursing may see its position. Hochschild was the first to adopt the term 'emotional labour' to describe not only care but also the conflict she saw as inherent in reproducing its 'private' (affective) manifestation within the 'public' (professional/ therapeutic) arena, where personal and emotional feelings have to be suppressed, or at least controlled. Smith (1992) argues that such a stance merely serves to perpetuate the traditional mind/body, feelings/tasks dichotomy, which a more modern and relevant interpretation (such as epitomised by Benner & Wrubel, 1989) seeks to integrate.

Smith's argument is persuasive and not without support. Indeed, such clear conceptual demarcations in caring by typologies appear somewhat untenable when related to practice (and especially when related to a hierarchical value system). Savage (1995), for instance, notes that caring in the public sphere, often conceived as inferior to that within the domestic domain, is often characterised by love and affection, while the domestic scene can be the site of violence.

The equation of love with caring here – and particularly with professional caring – is interesting, though not unique. Clifford (1995), in her review of the literature, describes caring as 'loving' in terms of providing support to others in need. And Smith (1992) herself, discussing Hochschild's 'emotional labour', sees emotions as the 'love' part of caring, which is in danger of being replaced by social distance when there is an over-concentration on physical tasks alone. Perhaps the most consummate argument for professional care as being compatible with the concept of love is provided by Campbell (1984, 1985). Basing his logic partly on the work of Halmos and the 1960s counselling ideology which viewed the exercise of therapeutic skills very much in the affective domain, Campbell (1984) argues that the love which is self-evident in informal caring modes, is actually central to the very meaning of care irrespective of context. Therefore any attempt to mark off a purely professional type of care through an overemphasis on competence will carry a danger of losing the essential characteristics of spontaneity and simplicity. Thus he sees professional care as actually a form of 'moderated love'.

There appears currently, then, to be support for the notion that care is an integrated, rather than dichotomous, concept, but with various manifestations. Kitson (1987), writing from a nursing perspective, articulates these ideas as they might apply to the discipline. Her interpretation sees both lay and professional caring as being characterised by the trust of the care recipient, commitment of the care giver, a belief in the promotion of the best interests of the recipient and the knowledge and skills of the carer. However, in professional caring these characteristics are further circumscribed by the contractual nature of the caring process, which makes it more complex. The usefulness of this model to nursing will be discussed after a consideration of Morse *et al.*'s (1992) remaining two identified dimensions of care.

Care as an interpersonal interaction

Morse *et al.* (1992) describe a 'mutual endeavour' between care giver and care recipient with both parties involved in, and enriched by, a communicative, trusting, respectful and committed understanding. In this respect, care as an interpersonal interaction is very much linked to both care as an affect (discussed above) and care as a moral imperative (discussed below). A number of other commentators and theorists make the same connection. Benner and Wrubel (1989), for instance, write about the carer being 'connected and concerned' with the clients, Savage (1995) about an 'attachment and emotional relationship' and Campbell (1985) about pastoral care as a kind of 'friendship' or 'relationship'.

This perspective would appear to be uncontentious as far as it goes. However, it could also be seen as somewhat limited, overly positive and as raising a number of issues if applied to nursing. First, although, as Clifford (1995) notes, the literature largely sees the process of caring as involving two people, Morse *et al.* (1992) raise the question of whether caring takes place within groups and, if so, whether its nature differs from that undertaken at the individual level. The question is not answered, but the authors do point out that caring theorists do appear to have ignored this issue, particularly at the family level.

Secondly, the literature on caring as a relationship does tend to assume this implies benefits to both parties involved, and the current language of 'partnership' and 'participation' within the new patient/provider relationship (Wade 1995) only serves to enhance this positive stance. However, Benner and Wrubel's (1989) work also points up the risks, vulnerability and stress which are corollaries of the caring relationship, while the conflict inherent in the 'emotional labour' described by Smith (1992) has already been mentioned.

Thirdly, and a further potentially negative characteristic which needs to be taken into account, is the element of power which is integral to a caring relationship. Campbell (1984, 1985), analysing the nature of caring professions, writes about the ambiguity in the notion of professional care, given that other people's ill health and social disadvantage are sources of power, status and income for those professionals. The odd juxtaposition of service and personal advantage, he argues, means one cannot totally ignore the charges put by Illich (1977) against what he saw as power-seeking 'disabling professions'. The point has not gone unnoticed by Savage (1995) in her review of the issues. Savage cites Hockey (1990) who comments that care, while rooted in the Christian concept of love, nevertheless coexists in uneasy proximity with the concept of control. Wade (1995) and Webb (1996), however, see the power factor in professional caring as perhaps more historical than current. Both allude to the traditional authoritarianism which has characterised the medical profession's relationship with clients, dominated as it has been by an emphasis on success in treatment. The so-called cure/care dichotomy, where care is more accepting of professional fallibility, is seen as a reaction to this.

Care as a moral imperative

The notion of care as a moral imperative is not unrelated to this last point. Indeed Webb (1996) explicitly argues that the ethical dimension has been largely ignored in the medical quest for professional certainty and success. So, too, Illich's 'disabling professions' might be seen as essentially amoral were it not for the imposition of ethical codes on their actions.

The need for such codes itself raises the question of whether any moral component to caring is, in any case, 'natural' to professional human endeavour. Benner and Wrubel's (1989) reading of the concept would suggest it is, when they describe it as meaning that 'persons, events, projects and things matter to people' (p.1). Similarly, Heidegger (1972), on whom Benner based much of her thinking, argues that it is through care or concern that people have their being in the world, while Campbell's (1984) 'moderated love' construct entails personal commitment beyond a contract and, therefore, one would suppose, irrespective of external sanctions. Titmuss (1970), on the other hand, who sees care as a type of altruistic 'giving', also regards men as not being 'born to give' and therefore needing to learn how. Clifford's (1995) point that personal motives may be dominated by a less than purely altruistic need to care seems to support this argument.

Steering a path between these tendencies is the view that caring is about the *way* things are done, rather than (or possibly as well as) *what* is done (Clifford 1995, Fealy 1995, Webb 1996). In other words, caring may be seen

as a disposition, and activities may be carried out in either a caring or uncaring way. The moral dimension here consists of the bases of judgements underpinning, and the consequences of, those activities (Fealy 1995), intended consequences being to do with some benefit to the recipient of care (Clifford 1995). If moral principles can be said to be concerned with this 'informed action' and with the related concepts of responsibility and accountability, as Fealy (1995) asserts, it can perhaps be seen why claims have been made for a moral component to professional caring in particular.

The final points to be made related to care as a moral imperative have more negative connotations. If caring is about disposition rather than activities *per se*, then activities which may otherwise be designated as 'caring' may need redesignating if carried out in a perfunctory or grudging manner (Webb 1996). This interpretation would have implications for all so-called 'caring professions' insofar as the claim to that label will depend primarily on the possession of a corporate attitude rather than particular skills and knowledge. A further 'negative' side to the moral dimension comprises some of the less attractive characteristics of care, particularly as they affect the carer, highlighted in the research. These include pressure, stress, unrealistic expectations and the burden of caring (Lea & Watson 1996) and may serve to offset the reciprocity in the caring relationship that is highlighted above.

In summary, the concept of care, as described in the literature, is seen as inclusive of a broad range of different, and often opposing, dimensions which include both generally 'positive' and 'negative' connotations. This inevitably makes its application to practice in any setting highly problematical, since it begs the particular identification of appropriate traits within the breadth of characteristics. In order to discuss whether nursing has claims to caring as an enduring and central feature, its own values need to be analysed for their compatibility with what has been highlighted regarding this ideal.

Caring and nursing ideals

One of the difficulties in isolating specifically nursing ideals is that they are often only described in terms of an assumed and accepted concept of caring itself, thus creating something of a tautological situation. Thus the Department of Health (DoH 1989) in its *Strategy for Nursing* noted that 'nursing is professional caring' and that 'the ideal is common to nursing, midwifery and health visiting and is central to their enduring appeal' (p.7).

This is reiterated in the Consultation on a Strategy for Nursing, Midwifery and Health Visiting (NHSE 1998), which emphasises the importance of retaining caring at the heart of nursing as the profession moves forward to develop new roles and adopt new priorities (e.g. adopting a public health approach, creating effective alliances and partnerships with other health professions and agencies to improve health promotion activities) in acute and community services. The consultation document cites the support of the white paper *The New NHS*, published in 1997, for nurses 'working across organisational boundaries to ensure continuity and integration of care' (p. 46). It goes on to say:

> 'Careful consideration needs to be given to ways in which this objective can be supported, not least because concern has been expressed that role development could result in the fundamental aspects of nursing, midwifery or health visiting practice being overlooked and undervalued. The public hold nurses, midwives and health visitors in high regard ... because of the quality of their caring. ... A key challenge is to ensure that the development of nursing, midwifery and health visiting roles commands public support and values the essential aspects of caring which are the very foundations of professional practice.'

(NHSE 1998)

Similarly, Coulon *et al.* (1996) found caring to be one of the recurrent themes in both a literature review and empirical research on 'nursing excellence'. Yet, despite this, Smith (1992) found in her own research that students complained that nothing was really said about caring during courses of educational preparation.

Perhaps one of the reasons for this is that nursing, like caring itself, is largely invisible and therefore 'assumed' rather than expanded on in many contexts. Savage (1995) noted this as a possible explanation for her observation that nurses have traditionally had difficulty articulating what is special about what they do, since 'often the highest art of nursing is making it look and feel as if people are not being nursed at all' (Preface). Paradoxically, however, she also noted that nursing's cost-effectiveness is often calculated on the basis of what is observable and measurable when visible. Clearly it behoves nurses at least to attempt to describe their work and the knowledge which underpins it.

Indeed, many nurse theorists have done just this. And in the debate one can see reflected the polarisation of views on theory development seen in the caring literature, which inevitably impacts on the values upheld. On the face of it, the reductionist, logico-positivist framework for explanatory analysis appears to be universally censured for its failure to comprehend the whole of nursing with its expert knowledge embedded in everyday 'unsanitised' practice (Benner & Wrubel 1989, Lawler 1991, Clifford 1995). However, what to construct in its place has remained a debating point, and has presented researchers with a problem. As Savage (1995) has commented 'there is no appropriate language to express the experiential, intuitive and creative dimension of nursing' (p.126).

A number of nurse researchers have turned, in seeking solutions to this dilemma, to the more inductive approaches. Benner & Wrubel (1989), for instance, followed the 'theory-from-practice' route in describing the primacy of caring in nursing, arguing that 'the phenomenological and feminist goal of making visible the hidden offers a view of the person which is an alternative to Cartesian dualism' (p.xii). Similarly, Lawler (1991) took a grounded theory approach in order to accommodate 'the body' within an academic study of the intimate and physical side of nursing practice. Savage's (1995) study of 'closeness' in nursing was built on an ethnographic framework which could take account of the experiential nature of much knowledge, while Allan (1996) used Watson's (1988) theory of nursing, with its phenomenological and humanistic basis, to enable students to identify 'carative' factors in nursing.

Yet, notwithstanding these credible and often highly acclaimed studies, the debate over how nursing theory (and therefore nursing values) are developed continues. Bradshaw (1995) echoes Henderson in describing nursing as being in 'total intellectual confusion' and offers a thoughtful, if rather damning, critique of the development of nursing theory over recent years. In particular, she questions the phenomenological approach of nurse researchers such as Benner, Melia and Robinson, to whom nursing practice is defined in terms of whatever it means to individual practitioners. If there is no one reality or universal theory, argues Bradshaw (1995), then what criteria can be used to judge someone's action, based, as it is, on intuition? What constitutes good practice and how can expertise be defined? This is the problem of scientific relativism.

However, the issue extends beyond this, according to Bradshaw (1995). The theory of pragmatism – truth derived empirically from practical activity – to which this allegiance to inductivism gives rise, is, she claims, inherently unstable, as it is difficult to decide what counts as knowledge. To Bradshaw, nurse theorists appear to have been forced to move to either the positivist-functional approach to building knowledge (such as Roper, Roy and Orem) or to the more interpretive position of Riehl and King. Either way, she argues, there is still a reliance on hidden assumptions, based on the supposedly universal and traditional 'common sense' view of nursing which, incidentally, patients also uphold. On this basis it is difficult to build up nursing theory at all.

Perhaps one way out of this difficulty in articulating nursing values, at least for the purpose of the present debate, is to look again at Morse *et al.*'s (1992) dimensions of caring and identify any reflection of them in the nursing literature, while acknowledging the paradigm or theoretical viewpoint from which the literature emanates.

Nursing as affective and/or therapeutic care

The integrated nature of care as outlined above and claimed by Kitson (1987) for nursing is perhaps more easily analysed in its major component parts. There is, for instance, prima facie evidence to support the notion of nursing as the embodiment of caring in its therapeutic guise, at least at some points in its history. Bradshaw (1995) and Clifford (1995) both comment that the traditional nursing practice of about 25 years ago very much emphasised its practical and physical components and a system of skill development based on clearly defined rules directed towards cure and much influenced by the medical profession. Menzies' classic analysis of nurses' use of defence mechanisms in order to maintain the distance this required, bears testimony to the sequel of this approach in terms of nursing behaviour (Menzies 1970).

More recently, recognition has been given to the 'emotional' side of nursing practice as an ideal emanating from the 'new nursing' movement (Smith 1992, Savage 1995). Smith (1992), whose concept of care based on the work of Hochschild has already been noted above, came to recognise this 'emotional labour' as integral to nursing through interviews with student nurses and patients in order to elicit their personal perspectives. In a similar respondent-focused study, Savage (1995) found that nurses interpreted their work in terms of an emotional 'closeness' which involved (often reciprocal) self-disclosure.

Yet, despite the frequency with which this care/cure debate occurs in the literature, often accompanied by analogies to the male/female and doctor/nurse divisions of labour (Webb, 1996), this is perhaps an oversimplistic way of analysing the distinctiveness of nursing as it moves easily from the one to the other (Webb & Hope 1995). Firstly, evidence from research which seeks a multiperspective definition of reality has found that nurses and patients/clients do not necessarily agree on priorities of value in nursing (Clifford 1995, Webb & Hope 1995, Webb 1996). In most reviews it appears that patients value technical skills more highly than nurses, who emphasise the emotional aspects, although Webb & Hope (1995) in their study found the reverse to be true. These authors offered possible explanations for their findings, such as the fact that technical aspects may be taken for granted by nurses, therefore not thought worthy of mention, or that their particular group of patient respondents were relatively young and not typical. However, in conclusion they argue that there may be a broad sympathy with the 'new nursing' ideals on the part of younger patients.

A second point to make is that, although a move to a more affective approach to care may be seen as progressive, liberating and more uniquely characteristic of nursing, it may also be more problematic. Savage's (1995) exploration of what the concept of 'closeness' means to nurses found that its more negative implications included unclear work boundaries, emotional cost, reduced group cohesion and a difficulty in demarcating feelings appropriate for the work situation and those which are more private. Smith (1992) also noted the anxiety-provoking nature of her study of emotional labour.

Thirdly, it is unclear whether values found to be relevant to one specialist area of nursing are necessarily applicable to all specialisms. Warelow (1996), while noting that 'empathy and emotional understanding through disclosure are already part of the established mandate of psychiatric nurses' (p.657), laments the dearth of information relating to care from other areas of practice which would enable some claim for greater universality of this dimension. Similarly, the work of Bignold *et al.* (1995) on 'friendship' as a viable construct in the work of specialist paediatric oncology nurses, revealed some interesting personal interpretations on the part of the nurses interviewed. However, the extent to which these findings can be generalised to the whole of nursing is debatable.

Finally, there is the potential problem that nursing theory, for all its sophisticated articulation of what nursing is 'ideally', may be out of tune with actual practice. Campbell (1984) provides an example of this danger in his comparison of the theories of Hall and Orem, who emphasise the 'being with' (affective) side of caring in nursing, with empirical research which has suggested that, in practice, nurses are either socialised into emphasising the physical tasks (Clark 1978) or, once qualified, actually prefer this aspect (Stockwell 1972). Campbell concludes his analysis with the comment that the wrapping up of simple ideas in scientific terminology can distance practitioners from humanity; real-life problems of, for instance, balancing closeness and distance which are encountered in practice, are overlooked by theories.

Nursing as an interpersonal interaction

There can be little doubt that the issues and problems surrounding the professional caring relationship in general, noted above, are equally applicable to nursing. Although as an ideal it is exalted in much of the nursing literature, the potential for stress and anxiety as a by-product of this relationship is the same as that occurring through the 'affective' component of personal human caring. At the same time, the use of power within the relationship cannot be ignored.

Bradshaw (1995) notes that the emphasis placed on skills ('doing to') in the nursing of the past undermined the notion of a personal relationship of the kind characterised, at least theoretically, in the 'new nursing' by a greater involvement on the part of the patient/client. This greater involvement is variously expressed in the literature as 'active participation' (Clifford 1995), 'partnership' (Webb & Hope 1995) and 'reciprocity' (Wade 1995, Webb 1996).

Yet, at the same time as the elevation of this ideal, a note of caution has been sounded by a number of commentators questioning both the actual existence, and the appropriateness, of such equality of relations in nursing. Bradshaw (1995) reiterates the dilemma put forward by Campbell (1984) regarding power inequalities in professional caring. In fact she argues that nursing could be seen as one of the 'disabling professions' itself if, extending her critique of the phenomenological view that there are no absolutes, it meant that nurses are kept as the experts, there being no criteria against which to challenge this. The argument is applied in particular to Benner & Wrubel (1989) who claim to base their work on the thinking of the philosopher Heidegger. For 'Heideggerian philosophy does not provide a basis for the relationship on which care for others depends and which is at the centre of nursing' (Bradshaw 1995, p.85). Instead, it inhibits the patient's selfhood and focuses on the nurse. Campbell (1984) himself makes the point that certain types of care, such as bodily care, which nurses engage in, could, like the care a mother gives to her child, lead to a means of control.

It could also be argued that nurse theorists who explicitly base their conceptualisation of nursing on a human relationship implicitly depict a relationship of inequality. Webb & Hope (1995), for instance, describe Travelbee's aim of the interpersonal process which is nursing, as being to 'influence' others, while Peplau's interpersonal relationship is seen as therapeutic ('doing to') and educative – a point also noted by Wade (1995). Teaching and education are, indeed, common features of nursing role descriptions (King, Orem, etc.) but do not imply a true relational equality.

As to whether this equality is, in any case, appropriate, Webb & Hope (1995) question whether, on the one hand, nurses want a close, non-hierarchical relationship with patients which could undermine their authority and trust, while Wade (1995) asks whether, on the other hand, all patients necessarily wish to be empowered. Clearly all nursing situations would not benefit from this ideal. Campbell (1984) points out that such mutuality which is characteristic of the mother–child relationship cannot be applied to nursing since the nurse is not the patient's mother, and to regard her as such demeans the patient. Another illustration of the point is made by Warelow (1996) who provocatively asks whether theorists would still encourage in-depth relationships between nurses and patients where the former were likely to be spat on, verbally abused or punched.

Nursing as a moral imperative

Much the same arguments as those pertaining to relationships in nursing can be applied to the moral dimension. The traditional view of nursing as a vocation, based on an ethical and spiritual framework (Bradshaw 1995) still claims some adherence from modern theorists and lay observers. Benner and Wrubel (1989) suggest nursing is 'viewed as a caring practice whose science is guided by the moral act and ethics of care and responsibility' (p.xi), while Smith (1992) found in her interviews with patients that nurses were still seen as angels of mercy, and nursing as a vocation.

However, as with the claim to relational mutuality, there may be an oversimplistic, and somewhat anachronistic, assumption underpinning these ideals. For instance, the question of whether a moral dimension is naturally inherent within professional caring may be asked of nursing. Fealy (1995) suggests that nurses act in an ethical way because, as members of a professional occupation, they are guided by codes and standards, indicating, perhaps, as did Titmuss (1970), that such behaviour is externally motivated.

A different line of reasoning is adopted by Bradshaw (1995), but the effect of questioning an inherent ethic of nursing is the same. Bradshaw argues that moral relativism is an inevitable consequence of the scientific relativism she challenged as a means to theory development. And one of the consequences is that the meeting of nursing needs will depend on who holds power. The issue of equitability, implicit in this reading of the issue, is also mentioned by Coulon *et al.* (1996), who found in their study that this concept was only mentioned as being an essential nursing characteristic by learner nurses. Their hypothesis that the more experienced nurses subsumed this into their practice subconsciously may be plausible, but also serves to reiterate the point made earlier about the difficulty of uncovering nursing practice knowledge.

Finally, the question of whether caring, as depicted for instance by the dimensions described above, is an appropriate ethical ideal in all settings and with all patient groups, is posed by Warelow (1996). Should the same ethical principles guide the nursing of a recidivist child molester, Warelow asks, as those appropriate to an acutely ill hospitalised patient? Perhaps not, though the different context does not necessarily preclude a moral dimension in general.

The ideals of nursing, then, are not easy to encapsulate. Even given a framework of caring dimensions within which to analyse these ideals, it becomes apparent that the notion of caring is itself very broad and that nursing at different times and in different situations embraces the spectrum of this diversity. This has been seen with regard to the diverse methods of theory development put forward in the literature, and in the way nursing has been depicted across the various continua – as instrumental or affective, as a formal or informal relationship, as inherently moral or externally sanctioned. Yet, notwithstanding this apparently 'elastic' and nebulous interpretation, it does provide something of a basis from which to build a picture of how nursing is viewed conceptually in the managerial age which characterises the latter part of the twentieth century. This basis will be the subject of the last section of this chapter.

Focusing the definition

The foregoing review of care and of related values in nursing suggests that, although the two are interrelated, nursing, as Clifford (1995) points out, cannot legitimately make territorial claims to the study of care, since other members of the health care team (and, indeed, those outside it) have an interest in this. In order, then, to make this observation 'usable' and to focus the preceding analysis, it is suggested that an integrative, rather than restrictive, approach be adopted, but that features which mark out the characteristics specific to nursing care, and those which make the general ideal relevant to a given situation, are highlighted.

The suggestion, put forward above, that care and nursing may be characterised by features at one or other ends of various continua is, in effect, challenged in the literature by a number of writers who put forward a case for a more inclusive frame of reference. This is perhaps especially apparent with regard to the 'instrumental' versus 'affective' elements of the concept. Bradshaw (1995) points out that even in the 1950s and 1960s, when the traditional view of procedure-based nursing held sway, Evelyn Pearce was writing of the science *and art* of nursing, and balanced the emphasis with an appeal to patient-centred care. Meanwhile Savage (1995) suggests that with the advent of the 'new nursing' the meaning of care appears to be shifting from a predominantly 'caring for' focus to a broader interpretation including both 'caring for' *and* 'caring about'. Moreover, the 'existential presence' which is a feature of the latter is very much also 'therapeutic' in its own right. Much the same point is made by Smith (1992) in her suggestion that caring as the emotional side of nursing is distinct from, but complementary to, and underpinning, the functional attributes of the ideal nurse.

This has given rise to some new phraseology within the nursing literature. For instance Clifford (1995) describes nursing as entailing personal involvement in helping those for whom the nurse is responsible and, within that role, meeting the needs of the whole person – including instrumental and expressive elements – from a humanistic perspective. This she terms 'formalised caring'. Campbell (1984) offers another term to describe the 'moderated love' as it is expressed in nursing care: 'in place of stereotypes [we must] consider the tension in caring between 'being with' and 'doing to' and explore the possibility that nursing offers a love which is *skilled companionship'* (p. 35 – my emphasis). The skill component is crucial to the interpretation here and implies a knowledge base which marks out the professional nature of caring. Finally, Webb (1996) seeks to reconcile the caring and curing elements within nursing practice to offset what she sees as the tendency to focus on one extreme or the other. To assist with this she promotes the coping model of Folkman and Lazarus (1980), integrating problem-focused coping and emotion-focused coping, as well as the different health professionals.

A similar harmonising of opposite trends has been advocated with regard to the relationship issue in nursing. Both Benner and Wrubel (1989) and Gilligan (1982) make the point that independence and autonomy, which are often seen as valued goals for both patients and nurses, are not the characteristic features of mature and balanced adulthood. Rather, a relationship based on interdependence should be the goal, which should mean that the problematical issue of professional power becomes an irrelevance. Bignold *et al.* (1995), on the other hand, opt for a more 'cautious befriending' model for their community paediatric oncology nurses. Their argument that total reciprocity in professional relationships is not appropriate means that, though a subtle form of control may be inevitable, this is preferable to the more overt power regimes of institutional care.

With regard to the moral debate, Benner and Wrubel (1989) neatly bypass the either/or issue (in this case related to the internal or external motivation to ethical behaviour) through two lines of argument. Firstly, instead of questioning whether altruism is the basis for caring, they contend that caring is the basis for altruism (implying that the very business of caring will lead to a certain attitude). Secondly, they point out that concern for others and self-interest are not necessarily oppositional, especially within their phenomenological world view where the person is defined in terms of his relatedness to others.

Fealy (1995) is of the opinion that it is the moral dimension which characterises professional caring in particular. This is because it combines the concept of caring and justice and is thus similar to Campbell's (1984) point about care expressing itself in the form of social justice, thus synthesising the personal with the political. Perhaps this goes some way to addressing the question posed by Morse *et al.* (1992) about caring for communities. However, there is obviously still much work in this area to be done.

Such, then, is the case for inclusive caring values as a feature of nursing. However, there are inevitably a number of intervening variables which will impact on this broad interpretation to influence the actual practice of idealised nursing. These will be explored in depth in succeeding chapters, but two broad themes will be briefly highlighted here as an illustration of how they fit in with the above integrative framework.

One major theme is to do with the nature of nursing knowledge, how this is used and passed on, and how it articulates with the theoretical perspectives of other disciplines and occupations. Savage (1995) suggests how nurses can use a knowledge base which is specifically nursing orientated, yet may comprehend both the physical and emotional dimensions which typify the breadth of the caring ideal. Nurses, she says, employ knowledge of a patient's experience of the body during 'basic' nursing and this represents an example of how nurses simultaneously 'care for' and 'care about' the patient. Smith (1992) meanwhile, makes a plea for this complexity in the nature of care to be reflected in educational curricula by way of integrating intuitive insights with systematic knowledge. Putting this knowledge into practice, argues Clifford (1995), should make use of the problem-solving approach much favoured by other contemporary occupations and professions. The nursing process of defining nursing problems and implementing therapeutic nursing interventions should mark out the unique nursing contribution within the caring focus.

A final example of this approach to nursing theory is provided by Lawler (1991) in her discussion of how nurses can best accommodate 'the body' within a nursing theory that does not rely exclusively on either positivist science or the 'irrational and emotional'. An understanding of the body, she argues, 'is to have a comprehensive, integrated, composite view of assumed rules ... how these rules influence and structure social relations, and how the body as a thing is part of lived experience, and how those notions are integrated into a more general system of social relations. Such knowledge, however, is possible only through experience'(p. 226). This forms the basis of her theory of 'somology', which takes account of the body (soma) and is about learning and knowledge (ology).

The other major theme – that of context – is very much in keeping with Lawler's view of nursing knowledge which she describes as 'complex knowledge and integrative in the context of particular circumstances' (Lawler 1991, p. 226). Context here can be taken to mean broad trends, such as the historical context noted above, where the skill and technique basis of nursing some 25 years ago (Bradshaw 1995) has moved to a more balanced focus today (Savage 1995). It could also mean the more specific context for individual nursing practices, acknowledged by theorists and researchers in their studies of nursing (e.g. Smith 1992, Savage 1995). These contexts and their implications are reviewed in detail in Chapter 8.

This consideration of idealised nursing has put forward a framewc which sees the concept as inclusive of a number of theoretical, therapeutic, relational and ethical dimensions, centred around the concept of care, yet also capable of a dynamism which makes it responsive to changing situations. Webb (1996) perhaps sums up this approach in her review of the literature on caring: 'caring is an interactive process which requires the carer to be responsive to the needs of the person cared for, the resources available and the context in which the care occurs. This involves skilled assessment, planning, action and evaluation of the implications and nuances of all these factors. Nurses have a word for this process – it is called nursing' (Webb 1996, p.962).

References

Allan, H. (1996) Developing nursing knowledge and language. *Nursing Standard*, **10** (50), 42–4.

Benner, P. & Wrubel, J. (1989) *The Primacy of Caring: Stress and Coping in Health and Illness*. Addison-Wesley, California.

Bignold, S., Cribb, A. & Ball, S. (1995) Befriending the family: an exploration of a nurse–client relationship. *Health & Social Care in the Community*, 3, 173–80.

Bradshaw, A. (1995) What are nurses doing to patients? A review of theories of nursing past and present. *Journal of Clinical Nursing*, 4, 81–92.

Campbell, A.V. (1984) *Moderated Love: a Theology of Professional Care*. Society for Promoting Christian Knowledge (SPCK), London.

Campbell, A.V. (1985) *Paid to Care? The Limits of Professionalism in Pastoral Care*. SPCK, London.

Clark, M. (1978) Getting through the work. In: *Readings in the Sociology of Nursing* (R. Dingwall & J. MacKintosh). Churchill Livingstone, Edinburgh.

Clifford, C. (1995) Caring: fitting the concept to nursing practice. *Journal of Clinical Nursing*, 4, 37–41.

Coulon, L., Mok, M., Krause, K.-L. & Anderson, M. (1996) The pursuit of excellence in nursing care: what does it mean? *Journal of Advanced Nursing*, 24, 817–26.

DoH (1989) *A Strategy for Nursing: a Report of the Steering Committee*. Department of Health, London.

Fealy, G.M. (1995) Professional caring: the moral dimension. *Journal of Advanced Nursing*, 22, 1135–40.

Folkman, S. & Lazarus, R.D. (1980) An analysis of coping in a middle-aged community sample. *Journal of Health and Social Behaviour*, 211, 219–39.

Gaut, D.A. (1983) Development of a theoretically adequate description of caring. *Western Journal of Nursing Research*, 5, 313–24.

Gilligan, C. (1982) *In a Different Voice: Psychological Theory and Women's Development*. Harvard University Press, Cambridge, Mass.

Heidegger, M. (1972) *On Time and Being*. Harper & Row, New York.

Hochschild, A. (1983) *The Managed Heart: Commercialization of Human Feeling*. University of California Press, Berkeley.

Hockey, J. (1990) *Experiences of Death: an Anthropological Account*. Edinburgh University Press, Edinburgh.

Illich, I. (1977) Disabling professions. In: *Disabling Professions* (I. Illich, I.K. Zola, J. McKnight, J. Caplan, & H. Shaiken). Marion Boyars Publishers Ltd, London.

Kitson, A.L. (1987) A comparative analysis of lay-caring and professional (nursing) caring relationships. *International Journal of Nursing Studies*, **24** (2), 155–65.

Larson, P. (1984) Important nurse caring behaviours perceived by patients with cancer. *Oncology Nurses Forum*, 11, 46–50.

Lawler, J. (1991) *Behind the Screens: Nursing, Somology and the Problem of the Body*. Churchill Livingstone, Melbourne, Australia.

Lea, A. & Watson, R. (1996) Caring research and concepts: a selected review of the literature. *Journal of Clinical Nursing*, 5, 71–7.

Leininger, M.M. (1981) The phenomenon of caring: importance, research questions and theoretical considerations. In: *Caring: An Essential Human Need* (ed. M.M. Leininger). Slack, Thorofare, NJ.

Menzies, I. (1970) *The Functioning of Social Systems as a Defence Against Anxiety*. Tavistock, London.

Morse, J.M., Bottorff, J.L., Neander, W. & Solberg, S. (1992) Comparative analysis of conceptualizations and theories of caring. In: *Qualitative Health Research* (ed. J.M. Morse). Sage Publications, Newbury Park.

NHSE (1998) *A Consultation on a Strategy for Nursing, Midwifery and Health Visiting*. Health Service Circular 1998/045. National Health Service Executive, London.

Orem, D.E. (1980) *Nursing: Concepts of Practice*. McGraw Hill, New York.

Savage, J. (1995) *Nursing Intimacy: an Ethnographic Approach to Nurse–patient Interaction*. Scutari Press, London.

Smith, P. (1992) *The Emotional Labour of Nursing: How Nurses Care*. Macmillan, Basingstoke.

Stockwell, F. (1972) *The Unpopular Patient*. RCN, London.

Titmuss, R.M. (1970) *The Gift Relationship: from Human Blood to Social Policy*. Allen & Unwin, London.

Wade, S. (1995) Partnership in care: a critical review. *Nursing Standard*, **9** (48), 29–32.

Warelow, P.J. (1996) Is caring the ethical ideal? *Journal of Advanced Nursing*, 24, 655–61.

Watson, J. (1988) *Nursing: Human Science and Human Care*. National League for Nursing Press, New York.

Webb, C. (1996) Caring, curing, coping: towards an integrated model. *Journal of Advanced Nursing*, 23, 960–8.

Webb, C. & Hope, K. (1995) What kind of nurses do patients want? *Journal of Clinical Nursing*, 4, 101–8.

Section 3
Nursing in a Managerial Age

Commentary: Managerial Influences on Nursing

This section develops the second theme identified in Chapter 1, by exploring how managerialism affects the practice and occupational development of nursing. In Chapter 4, Wells gives some detailed background about the rise of managerialism and the 'new public management'. The introduction of an internal market in health care in the UK is set in context to show that it was but one manifestation of the imperatives associated with managerialism and the management movement worldwide. Current policy proposals in the UK are directed at reducing the more competitive elements of the quasi-market in health care and promoting the role of professionals once more (DoH 1997).

Even so, the chief executive will have ultimate responsibility for ensuring the quality of clinical services, in conjunction with a lead professional. It remains to be seen how many nurses are appointed to such positions and whether forging such links between clinical and managerial roles will encourage equity or division. Wells argues that the growth and defining of 'professional management' as a distinct sphere is associated with a diminishing influence of nurses as managers and a reduction in their ability to control their sphere of practice. Subsequent chapters in this section take up these themes, arguing from specific example topics to demonstrate the continued management potential of nurses and the difficulties associated with achieving this potential within current organisational systems.

In Chapter 5, Edwards makes a clear case for insisting that the nursing role should be primarily a managerial one, with a specific responsibility for ensuring that appropriate high-quality care is delivered. Drawing on historical precedents and a critique of current research, she disputes the professionalist view that holistic caring can only be delivered personally by qualified nurses. Instead, she suggests that nurses should 'work through others' with well-supervised, unqualified but adequately trained, assistants delivering most of the hands-on care; the managerial role is critical in ensuring safety and quality.

In Chapter 5 Edwards focuses attention on two key issues: first, whether the patient experiences high quality, effective care, and second, the extent to which health care systems can afford to deliver exclusive and expensive nursing to everyone who needs it. By insisting that only qualified nurses can provide care, the profession has abdicated responsibility for ensuring that everyone receives it. This is a common accusation in another guise: by serving their own interests, the profession neglects to 'serve the public good' overall. However, this is no simple argument for a more dilute skillmix or simple, hierarchical delegation of tasks to be introduced. Instead, requisite variety and skill across the team remains central, to ensure that decision-making, accountability and control remains with the qualified nurse in a managerial role. Whether current health care systems will allow this to happen remains debatable, and is a theme taken up in Chapter 6.

In Chapter 6, Fitzpatrick and Redfern detail the different systems that are commonly used for organising nursing care, but echo Edwards' complaint about the lack of realism in the professional aspirations held by some nurses. In this chapter, managerial expectations are shown to be unrealistic as well; what is espoused is not necessarily what is practised. Thus, team nursing and primary nursing systems, implemented specifically as ways of ensuring that patients receive individualised nursing care, regularly fall apart when there are shortages of staff or of skills; then the old-fashioned, mechanistic management approach of task allocation is used as a fall-back position.

Drawing on recent research, including that of the 'demonstration' nursing development units funded by the Department of Health, the chapter reveals the 'critical minimum' specifications required to ensure that nursing can be delivered appropriately through a range of different ways of organising work. Unsurprisingly, regardless of the type of organisation, sufficient human resources, especially the need for adequate skill-mix and staffing levels, are essential prerequisites for individualised patient care. However, the tensions between meeting organisational goals and the needs of individual patients focus attention on the differences between nursing and managerial values. Unless nurses have the authority to lead their units, individualised patient care is unlikely to be achieved. The plea from this chapter is not, therefore, for one particular approach to be seen as the way forward, but for these critical minimum specifications to be implemented regardless of the type of organisation.

The final chapter in this section (Chapter 7) focuses on education, an important battleground between the so-called professionalists and managerialists in nursing. In nurse education, this division tends to be polarised along lines that emphasise either 'thinking' or 'doing'; these are regularly confounded with 'theory' and 'practice'. Thus, professional educators are stereotyped as wishing only to consider the abstract, unrealistic ideals, while the managerialists are accused of focusing only on tasks and 'cannon fodder' to replenish the numbers of staff queuing to leave the service in a state of stress and exhaustion.

Roberts and Barriball detail the long history of the so-called 'theory–practice' debates in nursing, but focus particularly on the major changes in nurse education that have occurred in the last ten years in the UK. This has been a period of great change in nurse education around the world; the USA began the move to a higher level of education for nurses, and the UK was only one among many countries to follow this trend. Two key issues are noteworthy. First, the move to higher education establishments was only partial, since the funding base remains firmly in the hands of NHS managers, being administered through educational consortia. Second, the changes were implemented by educationalists in response to requests from managers that they required thinking nurses with the capacity for intelligent action based on a reflective understanding of the nature of the system and its context.

The idea was to encourage the use of intelligence and initiative among professional nurses, as a way to help make the organisation more sub-stantially rational and effective in the longer term. However, as Chapter 7 shows, neither educational nor clinical systems have really adopted the new ways of thinking, nor become the kind of learning organisations that were envisaged by the architects of these educational innovations. It remains to be seen whether the expectations being raised by the 'New NHS' (DoH 1997) or the promised 'Strategy for Nursing, Midwifery and Health Visiting' (NHSE 1998) will bring about these changes. In the meantime, neither professionalists' aspirations to obtain control over preparation for entry to their profession, nor the organisational need for intelligent, critical thinkers who are able to respond flexibly in changing situations, are being satisfied. This unsatisfactory situation has led the UKCC to set up a commission of enquiry into nurse education; it is due to report towards the end of 1999.

Overall, this section unravels the detail of a great deal of managerially driven change within nursing. It highlights the major difficulties that arise in organisations based on the old-fashioned ideals of mechanical, hierarchical managerialism; however, it demonstrates the potential for the nursing contribution to be greatly enhanced if a more modern approach could be adopted.

References

DoH (Department of Health) (1997) *The New NHS. Modern, Dependable*. Cmnd 3807. The Stationery Office, London.

NHSE (1998) *Consultation on a Strategy for Nursing, Midwifery and Health Visiting*. HSC 1998/045. NHS Executive, London.

4 The Growth of Managerialism and its Impact on Nursing and the NHS

John S.G. Wells

Introduction

Since it was established in 1948 the National Health Service (NHS) has been subject to a number of managerial and organisational changes reflective, to a greater or lesser degree, of a concern for improved efficiency and effectiveness (Levitt & Wall 1989, Leathard 1990). Of recent changes the NHS & Community Care Act 1990 has been the most far reaching particularly in its impact on clinicians.

Apart from the purchaser/provider split and the creation of an internal market in health care, the most significant change initiated by the 1990 legislation was its emphasis on the role of managers (Gray & Jenkins 1995) and the explicit involvement of clinicians in the management process; in particular the relationship and accountability of clinicians for the management of limited resources, something which had not been a traditional part of their remit. This was implemented through the introduction of a market led 'managerialism'.

The concept of a 'market led managerialism', also called new public management, has at its heart notions of efficiency, performance objectives and cost effectiveness through the operation of competition and accountability for the use of resources (Hunter 1993, Gray & Jenkins 1995). As a result clinicians have been encouraged by their managers to take on a new public managerial perspective and responsibilities, in addition to their clinical duties, as a means of influencing decisions with resource implications (Gavin 1995). The result has been to draw many health professionals into the managerial life of organisations, beyond a pure clinical focus into aspects of the organisation as a whole. One example of this trend is nurses being encouraged and expected to take on a responsibility for marketing their organisation and its services to potential purchasers (Jowett 1996).

Inevitably there is concern among health care professionals about the impact this may have on professional values and interprofessional relationships (Eby 1994, Harrison & Pollitt 1994, Ham 1992, Wells 1996). It seems possible that there has been a change in the traditional self-image, perceptions, values and roles of individual health professionals (Wells 1995b). Moreover, health care professionals may find themselves in a position of role and value ambiguity, caught between meeting managerial targets and continuing to function within the parameters of their clinical traditions. This may lead them to act in ways which are aimed at managing their consequent anxieties rather than carrying out the tasks envisaged by senior managers and policy makers (Lipsky 1980). Whatever the reaction of clinical staff, it is plain that such an important shift in focus and autonomy has affected the culture and philosophy of the various professions, including nursing, within the NHS. In turn this affects the way the health care professions operate, not only within the NHS but also within society as a whole.

Although some research has investigated the impact of the Griffiths general management changes of 1983 (Strong & Robinson 1990, Gabe *et al.* 1994, Clark 1995), less attention has been paid to changes resulting from the NHS & Community Care Act 1990 (Connechen 1991). In particular, we know relatively little about how well prepared UK nurses are for their new managerial responsibilities and how this change in expectations in their role impacts on their values and focus (Wiggins 1997).

This chapter reviews the main local and national reforms to the management organisation of the NHS up to 1990. It discusses also the concept of managerialism and its influence on the management structure of nursing. These developments are examined in relation to the cultural and historical development of nursing and nursing management in the UK, so placing the 1990 reforms in context to allow an evaluation of their effects on nurses and the health service overall. The resource management initiative is considered to illustrate the changing relationship between nurses and the NHS. Finally, this chapter discusses the effect of these changes on the nurse manager, nursing practice and the nursing profession, with particular regard to nursing's involvement in the management process, its wider role within health policy and changes in the management and delivery of health care in the UK resulting from the Labour government's white paper *The New NHS: modern–dependable* (DoH 1997) and recent policy statements (e.g. DoH 1998).

Management tension in the early days of the NHS

The establishment of the NHS in 1948, with its emphasis on free delivery of treatment and care at the point of use, was a manifestation of a social, economic and political trend that developed in the first half of the twentieth century. This emphasised scientific principles and rational techniques of planning, implemented by large national bureaucracies, as an effective means of dealing with societal problems (Wolin 1961). This combination of science and management would enable, it was believed, rational use of resources and would greatly extend the ability of society to deal with problems that had been seen previously as intractable (Reed 1989). The nation's health problems were seen as compounded by competing parochial and historical vested interests which prevented rational planning and effective resource use. A national health service would enable services to be planned and co-ordinated (Strong & Robinson 1990).

Gray and Jenkins (1995) identified two features that characterised the 'new' state services, of which the NHS was the most prominent, in terms of organisation. These were a career-based structure of administration, and the organisation and delivery of services controlled by established professional groups. Thus within the NHS, management was largely a matter of administration and reconciling demands of policy with those of the professionals who delivered services, in particular the doctors.

Prior to the NHS the matron, always a nurse, exercised considerable managerial authority, but this was much diminished under the NHS structure. The writings of Nightingale and the work of early matrons, such as Eva Luckes at the London Hospital, established a wide management remit for this role in the hospital setting (Baly 1986). Most matrons were responsible for overseeing nursing care, management of all female staff (not just nurses but also groups such as domestics and radiographers), and also for managing nurse education. This gave them considerable power in relation to the hospital boards, who relied on them for advice and to take the lead on all non-medical matters (Abel-Smith 1964, Baly 1995). Such dominance fostered a maternalistic environment in which authority, hierarchy, clinical expertise and seniority of service were highly valued (Oroviogoicoechea 1996).

The administrative restructuring that took place under the NHS and, in particular, the appointment of administrators to the new hospital management committees, with no nursing equivalent at this level, reduced considerably the matron's remit, because administrators were given responsibility for non-nursing staff. This marked a shift in authority from seniority to technical competence (Schurr 1968). Consequently, the influence of the matron on the general life of the hospital slowly declined. This decline was compounded by the fact that the role of the matron varied widely from one hospital to the next (White 1985). The historical development of the matron's role had been individualist which resulted in matrons identifying with their hospitals rather than with their peers from other hospitals.

The new NHS structures resulted in considerable management tension between the matron and the administrator (White 1985). This led in turn, it has be argued, to a sense of insecurity for all nurses, which was manifested for many in defensive and negative attitudes to hospital management, which have persisted to the present (see for example Haywood 1968, Wilson-Barnett 1973). Perhaps in reaction to the decline of the all-encompassing power of matron, future nurse managers saw their remit as a narrow one, focused on professional issues and the management of the nursing workforce alone (Wilson-Barnett 1973). Taken together these factors may help to explain the failure of much of nursing management in the 1960s and 1970s to adapt from a model which was based largely on regimentation, seniority of service and the carrying out of orders (Duffield & Lumby 1994) to one that was more innovative, proactive and rationalist in approach.

A number of studies in the 1960s, 1970s and early 1980s demonstrated that nurses viewed management, nurses in management and the management role negatively. Haywood (1968) found numerous problems of understanding in the relationship between the nurse at the bedside and the nurse in management. Redfern (1981) found that ward sisters experienced conflict between their perception of their clinical role and the requirement to manage. Lathlean and Farnish (1984) found that nurses were alienated from management by what they perceived to be an industry orientated approach which they felt irrelevant to their clinical focus. This was reflected in the limited emphasis on management education for nurses in pre-registration training (Fowler 1984).

At nursing officer level Carr (1978) found a greater job satisfaction from teaching and clinical work than from management activities. However, a study of 100 nursing officers in Scotland in 1973 (Wilson-Barnett 1973) found that they spent relatively little time teaching or giving clinical support, despite the majority identifying advice giving, supporting staff and maintaining good relations with staff as important responsibilities. Such studies confirmed a general perception among nurses that those promoted on the basis of their clinical ability from sister to senior nursing officer no longer utilised their clinical expertise (Wilson-Barnett 1973). In turn this diminished the standing of these senior nurse managers in relation to their clinical colleagues and reinforced a negative view of the role of management in nursing. As we shall see, these attitudes and the lack of effective educative correctives were to have a serious impact on the ability of nursing to maintain both its management status and its influence on management policy in the 1980s and 1990s.

Managerialism

Though important managerial and organisational changes were implemented, until the 1960s the NHS remained largely unchanged in its philosophy and power structure (Leathard 1990). Organisational changes were concerned mainly with the provision and delivery of health care, for instance the expansion in the number of health centres (Leathard 1990). The ability of government to influence what actually went on within the various organisations (for example hospitals) was very constrained. Its role was confined largely to setting the overall budget within which activity could take place. This meant that the NHS was slow to respond to macro and meso policy initiatives. From 1948 to the mid-1960s changes centred on the need to streamline the service to aid accessibility. However, thereafter there emerged trends which, it could be argued, led to a dominant culture of 'managerialism' in the 1980s and 1990s and a more 'political' service.

Small (1989) characterises the dominance of managerialism in the NHS as the most important issue within the current analysis of health care delivery and its organisation. It is a concept associated with increasing the efficiency of an organisation through the synthesis of managerial expertise and corporate accountability (Small 1989). Roberts (1989) highlights the synergy of this development with the increased influence of the economic concepts of scarcity and finite resources within NHS policy-making circles. She describes the synthesis of these developments as rational managerialism.

The concept of rational managerialism came to the fore in reforms introduced by Sir Keith Joseph. These were an attempt to improve efficiency in the administration of the service overall, with an emphasis on planning as a means of better managing resources (Levitt & Wall 1989). The 1973 NHS Act was the first major reorganisation which affected the organisation as a whole (Ham 1992). Its principle aim was to streamline the service by bringing it under one authority and relating it to local government services. Underpinning this change was a belief that better management could be achieved through consensus management, multidisciplinary team work and giving medical staff a more explicit organisation-wide management remit.

The NHS Act 1973 introduced a tripartite arrangement of consensus management and collective responsibility consisting of doctors, nurses and administrators jointly managing at each level of the health service, but each managerially responsible for their own profession. The Act's significance for future developments was its emphasis on delegation of the managerial function downwards and accountability upwards (Ham 1992).

The trend towards bureaucratisation which this legislation represented was reflected in nursing. As White (1985) points out, the ward sister's role increasingly became an administrative one. Indeed, nursing's comparative lack of influence within the health service and confusion over its professional status, as reflected in its poor clinical career structure, led nurses to seek career advancement through seeking a more managerial role. The changes introduced to the career and management structure in nursing may be seen as part of this general trend (Department of State & Official Bodies 1968; DHSS 1972). The most important of these was the implementation of the recommendations that were contained in the Salmon Report (MHSHHD 1966) through the Mayston Committee (Cowie 1995).

Salmon and nurse management

Salmon's main aim was to increase the status of nursing and develop a rational career structure through establishing unit nursing officer posts, to provide authoritative front-line clinical leadership for the profession. Salmon established three functional forms of nursing management. The first, described as first line management, was concerned with organisational matters at ward level and focused on the allocation of tasks; this role was undertaken by ward sisters. The second, middle management, was charged with planning and providing resources for first line managers; this role was given to a grade of senior nurse. The third, top management, was charged with formulating and overseeing policy. This role was undertaken by directors of nursing at hospital and regional level.

It is important to note that nurses did not receive any formal training for their new administrative function. Salmon advocated front-line management training for nurses but this was never realised and those few formal courses that were established proved over time to be inadequate (Lathlean & Farnish 1984). Preparation for the management role followed what was essentially an informal apprenticeship model in which nurses were introduced to greater responsibility through their designated role on the ward (Pembrey 1978, Clark 1995).

Salmon's recommendations (MHSHHD 1966) became the bedrock of the nursing career structure until the changes of the 1980s. A number of research studies found that Salmon's original intention of providing a strong clinical front-line leadership role was not realised because unit officers became focused on their administrative activity (Wilson-Barnett 1973). Although those entering the nursing officer grades were often promoted on the basis of their clinical competence rather than any particular managerial ability (Owens & Glennerster 1990), their clinical focus was lost in their new role while they were ill-prepared for their administrative role. At the same time antagonism between the senior nurse and nursing officers often surfaced, fostered by the established nursing cultural tradition of rigid hierarchical attitudes which meant that accountability for decisions was pushed upwards (Owens & Glennerster 1990). Thus the relationship between nursing officers and those below them in the nursing hierarchy was often characterised by tension and alienation (Owens & Glennerster 1987).

Salmon reflected the general trend in the health service of the time towards increased status and authority for managers and the managerial role, a trend which was to achieve full expression in the 1980s and 1990s. However, nursing was ill-prepared to meet the challenges of the growth in managerial power and exhibited a degree of what might be termed 'schizophrenia'. Although the new management structure was seen as a way of increasing nursing's status, the negative attitude of most nurses towards management moved them in the opposite direction to the general trend in the health service. This resulted in lack of support among the nursing workforce for the development of a well-educated and a sophisticated nursing management cadre.

The result was that in the 1980s and early 1990s the nursing voice in management above ward level was muffled, if not extinguished. It is interesting to note that as the nursing managerial career structure has contracted in recent years there has been greater emphasis once more on the clinical expertise of nurses and on them developing an extended clinical role (Witz 1994); for example, nurses carrying out minor surgery and leading health promotion activities in primary care (Royal College of Surgeons 1998), and nurses manning a new 24-hour telephone help-line operating as a kind of triage of the airwaves for GPs (DoH 1997). Indeed, the 1997 white paper explicitly commits the government to facilitating the extended role of the nurse:

'The Government is particularly keen to extend the recent developments in the roles of nurses working in acute and community services. Expert nurses are taking on a leadership role, monitoring and educating nurses and other staff, managing care, developing nurse-led clinics and district wide services. They work across organisational and professional boundaries ensuring continuity and integration of care. The Government is committed to encouraging and supporting the development of nursing practice in these ways.'

(DoH 1997, p 46)

'New' managerialism in the NHS

The concept of rational managerialism incorporated into consensus and professional management systems proved popular with professionals. However, increasing concern over demands made on the NHS and its resources and, implicitly, the ability of the state to fund it during the late 1970s, coincided in 1979 with the election of Margaret Thatcher. She and her advisers identified consensus with lack of accountability for resource decisions and inherently inefficient (Hadley & Clough 1996). Thus the attitude of government became hostile to the established consensus management structure in the NHS.

A 'new' managerialism was established in the 1980s. Hadley and Clough (1996) describe it as 'scientific managerialism' or 'neo-Taylorism' (Taylor 1911). They characterise it as comprising an interplay of: productivity defined in economic terms; the necessity of a disciplined workforce; and a belief in the 'unique place of managers in planning, implementing and measuring production; and a belief in their unchallenged right to manage' (Hadley & Clough, 1996, p. 13).

This new managerialism was built around the idea of the 'professional manager', i.e. that management as a function was the same regardless of the organisation or persons to which it related. This was associated with a business orientation in which one person had to be seen to be in charge (Rawlins 1992) and was focused on commercial values such as cost-containment and customer satisfaction. This paradigm was reflected in a new managerial language which started to appear in the NHS; thus sisters and charge nurses were to gradually become 'ward managers' being 'accountable for managing resources efficiently' (Clark 1995). The new managerialism began with the implementation of the recommendations of the Griffiths Report (DHSS 1983) and reached its apotheosis in the enactment of the NHS and Community Care Act 1990.

The Griffiths Report

Sir Roy Griffiths, the Deputy Chairman and Managing Director of Sainsbury, was asked by the Conservative government to head up a small team charged with recommending changes to promote the efficient and effective use of the NHS workforce and resources. The recommendations of the subsequent report (DHSS 1983) centred around the management structure of the service at national, local and hospital level. Its main thrust was that an NHS Management Board should be established at the centre, with a chairman drawn from outside the civil service.

Ham (1992) argues that this proposal aimed to reduce the influence of the centre on day to day management and focus more on national strategic issues. This was strengthened further by the recommendation that general managers should be appointed at all levels in the NHS to provide an explicit focus for managerial accountability and with a remit to provide a dynamic leadership, motivate staff and promote change. The covert agenda, represented by general managers, was the introduction of the concept of accountability, effectiveness and cost-containment combined with an adoption of 'commercial' values and their application in the health care arena (Ham 1992). These last two, in particular, sat uneasily with the founding principles of the NHS and challenged the culture of professional and consensus management which had grown up within the service (Wilkinson 1995). Griffiths' proposals were explicit – doctors should assume a management accountability for their use of resources.

The government endorsed Griffiths' report and set about its implementation. Its emphasis on the accountability of one person for an organisation had a major impact on nurse management. The loss of the consensus model in favour of a general management one meant that directors of nursing became subordinates rather than equals in the management structure. As the 1980s wore on further changes, such as the introduction of clinical directorates, ensured the demise of the unit nursing officer. This is not to say that nurses did not occupy management positions. Many did. But they occupied these in the role of a 'manager' not as a 'nurse', and post-holders did not necessarily need to hold a nursing qualification. Some resistance to these changes was voiced by nurses, notably in a public campaign run by the Royal College of Nursing (Leathard 1990). However, within the councils of the decision-makers the argument had been lost, and the reorganisation of management structures failed to ignite public interest.

This development was not unique to the UK. In a number of countries grappling with managerial reform of health care, such as Australia, nurse managers were seen as neither important nor effective. Thus their numbers diminished and their responsibilities declined (Duffield & Lumby 1994). Oroviogoicoechea (1996) argues that this trend reflected an inability of nurses to articulate their traditional management function, although within the UK, at least, in the years immediately prior to these changes, many nurses were ambivalent about the need for a nurse manager at a senior level.

In some ways the Griffiths changes can be seen as a continuation of the reforms and developments of the 1960s to the 1970s, being part of an incremental growth in the influence of management and managers, coupled with a need for financial control and accountability. This is seen clearly in the increased involvement of clinicians, doctors and nurses in management, the Salmon Report (MHSHHD 1996) and the 1973 legislation, which gave increased prominence to managers and management by consensus. This theme was further elaborated by Griffiths, through raising awareness of the need for cost effectiveness and cost containment. However, where Griffiths broke with the past was in his attack on the concept of consensus management, and his introduction of the idea of the single, accountable manager. This shift led directly to the introduction of the NHS and Community Care Act 1990.

The 1990 reforms and the new public managerialism

The 1990 NHS & Community Care Act had, at its heart, the concept of a 'managerialism' rooted in a free market ideology and consumerism. It was based on a concept of health care organisation and delivery articulated by Alain Enthoven (1985) and his views on the relationship between health maintenance organisations (HMOs) and providers of primary and hospital health care in the USA (McKee & Laing 1993).

The white paper *Working for Patients* (DoH 1989a), which preceded the 1990 Act, was proclaimed by the government to be the biggest reform of the NHS since its establishment (Savage & Robins 1990). The impact of the reforms on the organisation, structure and culture of the NHS would seem to support this proposition (Ham 1992). The key elements of the Act were the development of an internal market, the delegation of power (and responsibility) to local management structures, separating the purchaser and provider functions, with money following patients, and the introduction of general practice funding.

The reforms reinforced a business mindset which informs much of the agenda and communication between the various bodies that make up the health service today (Paton 1996). The price of these changes was that the government's ability to control events was weakened, although it was still held accountable by the electorate for provision of care. The government needed therefore an alternative means of control to the old central command structures.

Managerialism, and what is described as the 'new public management' (Hunter 1993), having challenged the traditional professional ethos and encompassing financial management, can be seen to have met this need for control. The new managers became the central point of contact between politicians, the health professions, purchasers and patients and became a significant factor in the delivery and planning of health care (Gray & Jenkins 1995). The ultimate loyalty of new managers to the centre was secured by the short term nature of their contracts of employment (Wells 1995a). This new model of health services management emphasised firm decision-making, autocratic and independent management, maximum accountability and responsibility toward the goals of cost-effectiveness and tight budgetary control. This was reinforced by the need for health services to be competitive at all levels, and to be aware of the 'political' dimension in decision-making and its impact (Wells 1996).

McKee and Laing (1993) argue that the significance of the 1990 reforms lies in their interaction with changes introduced in 1984. General management strengthened the lines of accountability to the government at all levels for individual decisions, while the 1990 changes enhanced the ability of government to direct and control professionals and health care through:

> '... introducing the sanction of loss of revenue if providers fail to offer what purchasers want, placing purchasers at arms length from providers and accountability to the government. The effect has been to shift the balance of power over who should provide what sort of services away from health professionals in provider units.'

(McKee & Laing 1993, p. 14)

Thus the drive for increased efficiency and the growth of managerialism had, as an implicit agenda, the intention to increase the degree to which the centre could exercise control over clinicians' (particularly doctors') independence of action in relation to their use of resources. This agenda was articulated first in what became known as the resource management initiative (RMI).

The resource management initiative

The RMI was implemented in six pilot study centres. Its main purpose was to increase the responsibility of primarily doctors, but also nurses, for the management of resources by delegating responsibility for the management of a clinical budget to clinical teams within the hospital. The assumption was that by giving these professions a formal management role in resource allocation decisions, they would become more conscious of the resource implications that flowed from their clinical decisions (Keen & Malby 1992). A subsidiary purpose of the RMI was to increase the power of managers to influence service delivery. This would be achieved by establishing more comprehensive information systems on clinical activity, thereby enabling managers to negotiate workload arrangements with these clinical teams when allocating their budget (Ham 1992).

To facilitate the RMI the hospital organisation was divided into clinical directorates, each headed by a clinician, usually a doctor, who was supported by a business manager and a nurse manager. These directorates became, and have become, independent units with an identified budget, accountable for their particular patient group, their staff and supplies and some common services from the hospital. An evaluation of the initiative showed that units were more costly to set up than was envisaged, and the process of involving doctors was difficult and time consuming. Also there were few tangible benefits for patients, and better value for money was not achieved (Ham 1992). However, the staff involved appeared to favour the directorate structure because it gave them a greater sense of purpose and fulfilment (O'Kelly 1989).

Although the research findings were far from favourable, the RMI was adopted throughout the NHS. Indeed, the government re-emphasised the importance it attached to the concept of clinical accountability, and involvement, in the management of resources encompassed by the RMI:

'Those who take decisions which involve spending money must be accountable for that spending. Equally, those who are responsible for managing the service must be able to influence the way in which resources are used. ... the Government remains committed to introducing modern information systems to support both clinical and operational functions in hospitals.'

(DoH, 1989a, pp. 7–16)

Resource management and its impact on nursing

Keen and Malby (1992) carried out a research study of the impact of the RMI on nursing power and influence and the practice of nursing in the six pilot sites in which it was introduced. This study found that the Griffiths report (DHSS 1983) had led to many senior nurses losing their management function at the executive level and being given advisory and consultative roles to hospital management boards. The study found that nurses at senior level were poor at playing the 'management game', and that their power was weakened, especially if their director of nursing held an 'advisory' role on the board (Keen & Malby 1992).

It had been expected that the introduction of improved information systems and, in particular, the use of information technology, would enhance greatly both the quality and efficiency of nursing care. The RMI pilot study introduced computers into wards to collect and collate data concerned with patient dependency and nursing workloads, and to develop standardised care planning. The expectation that computerisation would save nurses' time, so enabling them to spend more time on direct patient care, was not met. Indeed the converse was true. There was also little evidence to suggest that the computerised data was used to revise ward staffing levels or to improve the quality or efficiency of care delivered. The information system proved to be inflexible in that it could not incorporate different nursing models and practices. In fact in wards that had developed their practice on contemporary nursing philosophy and theory, which promoted partnership with the patient, it was found that practice was compromised (Keen & Malby 1992). However, ward sisters favoured the RMI because they felt it improved relationships with ward consultants, led to more collaborative care planning, and promoted multidisciplinary audit (Keen & Malby 1992).

Overall, the evaluation of the RMI in the six pilot sites highlighted that nurses found it difficult to articulate specific skills that they had to offer to their medical and management colleagues in the area of resource management. According to Keen and Malby (1992):

'Their inability to respond to the management challenge of RM (has) left them severely handicapped in contributing to decision making above ward level.'

(p. 869)

The legacy of nursing attitudes to management in the first 50 years of the NHS would seem to have had an impact. Nurses were found unprepared to operate in an environment that demanded they think beyond professional/clinical issues. Consequently their ability to affect the overall health agenda at local and national level was limited. Their diminished status was confirmed by the new management structures failing to guarantee their position as of right. Indeed, at board level the nursing advisor role was usually combined with some other, such as director of quality assurance, as if the presence of a nurse on the board needed some justification outside their professional competence.

From the above discussion it is clear that nursing management beyond the ward level was not strengthened by the RMI; indeed it could be seen to have weakened it. At senior management level it appeared to confirm the view that a specific nurse management post was superfluous, whilst at ward level the nurse manager's closeness to budgetary responsibility compromised both their clinical autonomy and the idea of the patient as a partner. The RMI can be seen as a transitional stage in the development of the market in health care that was introduced in 1990 (O'Kelly 1989). It also introduced explicitly into the professional culture of nursing, managerial concepts of resource efficiency, resource accountability, and systematic information gathering through activities such as audit. Further, it legitimated at least in part, managers managing and controlling professional activity. The RMI therefore confirmed the culture of the new management ethos in the NHS. It is to this new culture's relationship and impact on the culture of nursing that we now turn.

The importance of organisational culture

The concept of culture, its influence on the behaviour of individuals or groups, and how it changes have long been recognised by the disciplines of history and social anthropology as an important area of study, although how culture is defined varies widely (La Monica 1990). More recently other disciplines, including nursing, have taken an interest in this concept (Duffield & Lumby 1994, Suomin *et al.* 1997). In particular, managers and management theorists have been interested in those facets that make up organisational cultures and their weltanschaung – set of shared beliefs, values, attitudes, traditions, language, rules, behaviours and ways of doing – and how these can be influenced or changed to achieve greater efficiency and other managerial goals (for example Checkland & Scholes 1992, Drucker, 1993, du Gay 1996). The general orthodoxy in management theory is that a strong, cohesive organisational culture is essential to an organisation if it is to be productive and effective (La Monica 1990).

Health managers' pre-occupations during the 1980s and 1990s with such issues as mission statements, organisational restructuring, creating a corporate identity, total quality management and so on, often appeared trivial and caused some negative comment among health professionals (Oni 1997). However, these preoccupations highlight the importance attached by managers to shaping the function of health care professionals and the context in which they work and from which they draw much of their professional identity. Health care reforms resulting from the NHS and Community Care Act 1990, in particular the creation of an internal health care market, were seized on by managers to create an environment in which professionals would internalise concepts of the corporate well-being of their organisation, such as resources and market share, in their approaches to patients and commissioners of services (Wells 1994).

The importance attached by managers to the shaping of the organisational culture is understandable when one looks at the functions culture serves within an organisation. It provides a means of: passing down expected behavioural norms to personnel; establishing commitment to a particular set of values and philosophy; directing individual and group activity towards desired rather than undesired behaviours; and increasing organisational effectiveness (Martin & Siehl, 1983). Health service managers recognise that achieving a positive organisational culture is important if the objectives set for them either by government or commissioners of health care are to be achieved.

Cultural conflict with nursing

It is significant to note that aspects of organisational culture are often points of conflict between managers and NHS personnel, such as nurses (Ackroyd 1995). This is because the traditional culture of the NHS was and still remains largely one based on roles, characterised by one author as 'tribes' (Rawlins 1992), such as doctors, nurses, occupational therapists. The new management within the NHS seeks to change this culture to one based around task or specific objective rather than role. This is because contractual reimbursement relates to tasks completed, for example numbers of hip replacements, rather than the processes by which they are achieved. This change from a role to a task culture presents difficulties for nursing, particularly because the profession over the past 20 years has been concerned with developing holistic rather than task-based practice.

The 1997 white paper (DoH 1997) does not change this broad managerial agenda, rather it refines it by setting up a performance framework which measures service efficacy as a whole. This framework comprises three areas for action:

- National standards and guidelines achieved through national service frameworks and a National Institute for Clinical Excellence
- A drive for high quality services at local level through explicit quality standards in long-term service agreements involving health authorities, trusts, primary care groups and others, and through a new system of clinical governance
- The Commission for Health Improvement set up to oversee the quality of clinical services and to help tackle shortcomings

The white paper confirms the desirability of cultural change by empha-sising the need for professional audit groups to gather information on the clinical performance of individual clinicians (Burns 1998) for purposes of comparison. Much emphasis is placed on clinical governance which involves members of different health care professions working together to set and monitor standards and trust chief executives taking responsibility for their implementation. Clinical governance may serve to both dis-courage tribalism and further enhance the power of managers over the clinical agenda within the hospital setting. This is because the monthly reports that this system will be expected to produce will enable the trust to be judged on whether or not it has met its contractual obligations as set out in the 'service agreement'. Thus the focus of this assessment will remain on fulfilling service agreement tasks.

It has been argued that nursing culture in the UK, its values and the way it organises its activities, reflects general economic and social trends in the wider society (Bevis 1983). If this is true then it would seem that the nursing environment over the last 50 years has been influenced by the development of welfarism and its ultimate expression in the dominance of the NHS in health care. Bevis (1983) describes the development over this time of a nursing culture which encompassed 'humanistic' values. These were incorporated formally within the structure of nurses' working conditions when the Mayston Committee (DHSS 1969), following the principles of the Salmon Report (MHSHHD 1996), introduced directors of nursing with responsibility for nursing services and, in so doing, gave nurses influence over the provision and management of the nursing resource. This development was accompanied by improvements in nurses' pay and conditions. Equal pay for male and female nurses was established, working hours were reduced and holiday entitlement improved. In addition, nur-sing staff were no longer required to live in hospital accommodation and they could marry without fear of jeopardising their career (Leathard 1990).

Accompanying these more liberal conditions was increased emphasis on professionalism of nursing, with the first university courses in nursing established in London and Manchester. In addition a humanistic approach was emphasised in the approach to care, where value was placed on the concern of the nurse for the patient as an individual person in the context of his family and community (a holistic perspective). An example of the growth in influence of these values and beliefs in nursing may be seen in the introduction in 1982 of a new training syllabus for mental health nurses (GNC 1982) which emphasised the importance of interpersonal skills and relationships in the process of care between nurse and patient.

Clay (1987) argues that in the 1980s this humanistic value system had existentialist principles added to it. He characterises these as the belief that the patient has freedom of choice. This means that they have the right to reject the advice and directions of health care professionals. The new emphasis is on caring, with the nurse first and foremost accountable to the patient (Clay 1987, p. 28). This may be seen also to reflect the development of consumerism within society in the 1980s (Harrison *et al.* 1992). The emphasis on purchaser and provider concepts in the NHS and the Patients' Charter (DoH 1991), detailing standards that the patient as customer could expect, in 1990 was part of this general trend within health care (Harrison *et al.* 1992, Hadley & Clough 1996) and the 1997 white paper (DoH 1997) suggests that this trend continues.

Although the development of practice theory within nursing emphasised humanistic principles, translating them into the reality of practice proved difficult and contributed to the now well known cliché, the theory–practice gap. The truth was that much of the nurse's role up to the 1980s, whether in clinical or managerial work, remained task focused and submissive to medicine and administrative structures (Salter & Snee 1997). This resulted in an overall culture of conformity within established structures and reinforced the public's view of nurses as being task-centred and subordinate to doctors. This stereotype provided nursing with a passive yet saintly identity which discouraged challenge to the status quo (Carpenter 1980), perhaps summed up by one doctor's description of a district nurse as 'the angel at sunset' (Wilson-Barnett 1988). The stereotyping of nurses helps to explain, at least in part, the relative disregard of the nursing profession by government, civil servants and professional administrators when developing policy (White 1985, Duffield & Lumby 1994); the introduction of general management in 1983 is a good example of the interests of the profession being ignored.

It may be argued that this traditional lack of regard of nursing from outside the profession was a driving force behind the search for a recognised professional identity. Nursing consciously followed a policy from the mid 1950s on, led by the Royal College of Nursing, to establish professional credibility (White 1985). This policy identified clinical autonomy as a key component of professionalism and thus inevitably viewed the managerialism of the 1970s and 1980s as a threat and, implicitly, incompatible with nursing (Porter 1992). However, whether or not nursing is a 'profession' proved to be a thorny issue, not least for nurses themselves (Porter 1992). Although nurses often describe themselves as professionals they have problems taking on some professional attributes. For example, the concept of professional accountability, as established by the United Kingdom Central Council for Nursing, Midwifery and Health Visiting (UKCC), the statutory governing body for nursing, remains one which nurses continue to find a challenge and threat, being used to relying on the persona of the doctor to shield them from external questioning (Evans 1993).

Further uncertainty may be seen with regard to the debate as to whether or not nursing should focus on the development of specialism or be generalist, and whether it should widen or narrow the entry gate (Porter, 1992, Wilson-Barnett & Beech 1995). This debate complements much nursing policy literature with regard to the rise of managerialism in the 1980s, which is seen as anti-professional, particularly in relation to clinical accountability, and by implication incompatible with nursing values (Porter 1992).

Thus in the 1980s, while managers came to see work in terms of tasks to be achieved, nurses no longer conceptualised their work in such terms, though often the reality was that it remained task focused. Nursing's ability to meet the challenge posed by managerialism in the 1980s was hampered by its unclear self-identity, combined with belief in a model of professional expertise and the role of the nurse as a holistic carer (Benner 1984), which did not match the concepts of the new management construct of health care. An example of how these differing conceptions of role and function caused real tension between the new management culture and the cultural values of nursing may be seen in the clinical regrading of nursing staff which took place in the late 1980s and its subsequent impact in differentiating management function from clinical function. This provided managers with an opportunity to re-orientate and reshape the nursing workforce's profile, but created much disquiet and conflict among nurses.

The regrading exercise

The mid 1980s, as far as nursing was concerned, were a time of industrial strife and discontent. The Royal College of Nursing had fiercely opposed the Griffiths' general management reforms which had taken place in 1984. It saw them, correctly, as a threat to the managerial influence of nurses that had been established within the NHS following the Salmon Report (MHSHHD 1966). The failure of this campaign left nurses feeling undervalued, with a growing perception that a career structure vacuum was in the making. This became coupled with discontent about pay and conditions among nurses and growing irritation over the government's failure to implement reforms in nurse education. The government attempted to diffuse this discontent by establishing an independent pay review body in 1984, implementing the Project 2000 (UKCC 1986) educational reforms in 1996 and, most significantly, establishing a new clinical grading structure for nurses in 1988 (Cowie 1995).

The new clinical regrading structure, as articulated by government and the professional nursing bodies, was designed to reward nurses who had achieved a high degree of clinical competence and responsibility, something which the changes wrought by Salmon had been consistently criticised for failing to recognise. However, the grading structure included both qualified and unqualified staff in a grading continuum and, in fact, the actual criteria applied often meant that nurses were rewarded for their level of responsibility, that is their management function, rather than their clinical competence. Thus, for example, many midwives were given the lowest professional grades (i.e. grade D). The result was that there were many local disputes during the implementation of the grading structure and some of these were not settled until the early 1990s (Gavin 1995).

Gavin (1995) has pointed out that clinical grading was, and is still, used to institute skill mix reviews in which the number of clinically qualified staff as a proportion of the workforce was reduced. Because the grading criteria are related mainly to functional responsibility, the regrading exercise served to facilitate the concept of professional managerialism in nursing; to be awarded a management grade of F or above does not (at least in theory) depend upon holding a clinical qualification. For example, the Audit Commission (1991), reporting on the management of the nursing resource, separated the concept of the nurse manager from that of the ward sister, though it is clear within the report that both are ward based. They differentiated these posts on the basis that the former manages the budget and the resources while the latter deals with day-to-day clinical decisions. Furthermore, because of the increased costs associated with the higher grades (grades H and I), managerial responsibility has been located at a lower grade (grade G), with few, if any, higher professional grades between this grade and the hospital board (Gavin 1995).

The Audit Commission (1991) endorsed the desirability of this structure from a financial point of view by equating what it described as a 'flat' management structure within nursing with a reduction of management costs. Indeed one of the notable features of management cost cutting that took place in the 1990s was that costs were saved through a reduction in the number of nurse managers and senior nurse clinical specialists as opposed to other types of managers (Hancock, 1996). This again seems to confirm the low regard in which the nurse as a manager seems to be held. For example, a recent study on senior executives in the NHS commented on the lack of representation of nurses in senior positions at both trust and health district level (Dawson *et al*. 1996). However, this may change as a result of the 1997 white paper (DoH 1997) because of the important role for nurses in clinical governance and in the new primary care groups which will be central to commissioning and overseeing health care delivery (DoH 1997, Maynard 1998).

Management and the nurse manager

From previous sections of this chapter, it is clear that changes over the past 25 years have had and will continue to have a profound effect on nursing. Nowhere is this better demonstrated than in the role of the ward manager. Up to the changes in the 1980s and 1990s the exclusive focus of the ward sister or charge nurse, as they were known, was the clinical management of staff. However, it is now very different. The clinical nurse manager is defined as the first level of management, that is the closest of all levels to the nursing workforce and patients. He or she is identified as crucial to the organisation's ability to meet organisational aims and objectives and quality assurance targets and provides the link between senior management and employees. Participation in hands-on care is not seen as part of the clinical nurse manager's function. In fact it could be seen as a distraction from their primary role of managing a service. It is now accepted that individual nurses should be professionally accountable for their practice. This means that the clinical nurse manager's liability for the professional practice of others is limited, although they do have continuing accountability for the ward or unit as a whole. The clinical competence of the nurse manager, though seen as relevant, is increasingly identified both by junior nurses and management as not of primary importance. Therefore one needs to ask what is the significance of the clinical nurse manager's position and what does it encompass?

Various studies have identified changes to the management role of the clinical nurse manager. One of the most striking changes has been in job title from 'sister' (or charge nurse) to 'ward manager'. This change in terminology carries implications as to where their focus now lies, in particular their responsibility and accountability for the administration of a ward budget (Matthews & Whelan 1995, Yassin 1996). Linked to this are two further activities, that of responsibility for maintaining standards of care, particularly in relation to ward audit (Cowpe 1995, Matthews & Whelan 1995) and sharing in the corporate responsibility for managing the service as a whole (RCN Management Association 1989, Cowpe 1995). All this needs to be demonstrated through the ability to efficiently plan and manage the ward and all those, other than medical staff, who work in it every day. Another significant break with the past is that, whereas most ward sisters had permanent contracts of employment, many ward managers have time-limited contracts, usually three years in the first instance, which are renewed subject to satisfactory performance (McSweeney 1991).

The approach of the Labour Government to the health service and its governance appears to only change the mood music in this regard, since it is as determined as its predecessor to emphasise effective and cost efficient outcomes combined with accountability and penalties for non-performance. Although the government talks of a return to a national pay framework it does not stress national conditions, but emphasises the importance of flexibility to reflect local conditions. Furthermore, the importance placed on clinical governance and comparative clinician performance data will continue to foster a highly pressurised practice environment for ward managers dominated by the requirement for careful resource management (DoH 1997). The psychological stress produced is likely to be exacerbated further by government proposals to introduce legislation requiring clinicians to deliver high quality care. The requirement to meet potentially conflicting demands is likely to lead to ever greater levels of psychological stress for nursing staff and increases the risk of 'burnout'. The demand to meet potentially conflicting priorities has been found to be associated with burnout among clinicians and management in mental health teams (Onyett *et al.* 1996).

These circumstances of the ward manager's employment conditions may have a number of effects on their practice. There may be a tendency by some ward managers, for example, towards a dominant rather than an inclusive style of management (Wells 1995a). However, the most significant effects probably arise from the accountability of the ward manager for managing limited resources. In short, their focus has changed to one of conservation of resources rather than patient care alone, thereby changing the nature of their relationship with nursing staff and patients. The question frequently asked of the ward or unit manager is, 'Did you end the financial year within budget?'. To be seen not to do so reflects badly on the ward/unit manager and, in view of the nature of their employment contract, becomes an important personal and career issue. Thus when resources become strained one is more likely to find the ward manager arguing for less patient throughput than for more money to meet patient demand (Wells 1994).

Nursing practice in the era of managerialism

In the field of clinical practice the managerial ethos may also be felt. *A Strategy for Nursing* (DoH 1989b) emphasised 'evaluation of interventions to change the traditional boundaries of clinical and professional practice' (DoH, 1989b, p. 13) and its acknowledgement of the cost imperative in shaping service delivery is a clear indication that the management preoccupation with resource conservation is a dominant determinant of clinical nursing. The strategy states that:

> 'Management is about taking responsibility for achieving the objectives of an organisation, within a framework for the delivery of agreed services from available resources.'

> (DoH 1989b, p. 27)

The 1997 white paper (DoH 1997) appears to endorse this conception of management which entered the NHS with the 1974 reforms and found explicit expression in the resource management initiative in the 1980s. The white paper states that the principles of corporate governance are to be extended systematically into the clinical community. In other words, managers alone will no longer be held accountable for a trust's performance – all staff will be held responsible.

Further, the white paper's emphasis on the role of primary care groups and, in particular, on GPs and nurses having a direct and wide commissioning role and control of resources, identifies the clinician clearly not only with responsibility for the use of resources but also with balancing competing claims arising from clinical/resource decisions. As Maynard (1998) points out, the government intends to apply a capitalisation formula to primary care and create a whole new management structure within primary care. Thus a government initiative that may appear to give clinicians autonomy and enhance the role of nurses will also, in fact, further control clinical behaviour and distance central government from the consequences of its decisions. The thrust of the Labour Government's policies, as with those of its predecessor, remains a managerialist one which emphasises efficient use of resources. For example, the Health Action Zones established in 11 areas of the UK from April 1998 (DoH 1998) aim to ensure full integration and collaboration between health, social and voluntary agencies to deliver health care at the lowest possible cost (Harrison & Pollitt 1994).

The current management agenda which is concerned with achieving efficiency, throughput and demands for evidence and information, and the restructuring of clinical practice that this often entails, have an important impact on clinical nurses. Fox (1992) argues that the rise of day surgery has diminished the role of nursing within this field. Wiggins (1997) describes how nurses in one surgical unit, though valuing holistic individualised nursing care, accepted and to some degree internalised the management view that such an approach in a resource limited service was not efficient or cost effective. As a result care in the unit was task orientated and routinised.

It seems likely that managers' focus on achieving goals and breaking down activity into its smallest elements for the purpose of costing is likely to lead to task-focused nursing practice. Further, since managers must be concerned with achieving objectives at the least possible cost, it is inevitable that nurses will be asked to expand the scope of their professional practice in some areas and reduce it in others. An example of this can be seen in the discussion surrounding the appropriate use of nurses to replace junior doctors (Maynard 1997b) and the expansion of unqualified support workers in mental health care (Johnson *et al.* 1997). Indeed, the Audit Commission (1991) has questioned the value for money of employing qualified nurses.

Nursing is particularly vulnerable in this respect because nurses comprise the largest proportion of the health care workforce and account for 47% of NHS expenditure (Hancock 1997). It is likely therefore that many of the tasks nurses carry out at the moment will be undertaken by non-nurses in the future (Healthcare 2000 1995, Salter & Snee 1997). Further, nurses are now expected to participate in developing and maintaining the corporate image of their employing organisation and routinely ask patients if they are satisfied with their care to ensure that complaints are minimised (Beecher & Couchey 1997).

Spurred on by the managerial agenda, evidence-based practice and clinical governance are now the watch words within nursing (Kenrick & Luker 1996, Maynard 1997a). It is ironic therefore that so much of managerial practice lacks a strong empirical base (Hunter, 1996). Indeed, a study highlighted this factor as one of the stumbling blocks in research utilisation among district nurses (Kenrick & Luker 1996). Nevertheless, nursing care has to demonstrate both cost effectiveness and relevance to corporate goals, through such management reporting activities as performance measurement (Dennis 1997). The emphasis within nursing on research-based practice is no longer concerned with an agenda of patient care alone but also with cost-effective nurse-led patient care (for example see Hancock 1994).

Nurses have been forced to justify their worth as a professional group within the health service on managerialist rather than purely professional terms. Thus when commentators question the cost-efficiency and cost-effectiveness of nursing (for example, Roberts 1996) the Royal College of Nursing responds by citing the results of an evaluation of nursing practice by Carr-Hill and colleagues at the Centre for Health Economics at the University of York (Carr-Hill *et al.* 1992) which found that a skill mix of highly qualified nurses provided better patient care than a skill mix of lesser qualified nurses, so providing evidence for the cost-effectiveness and cost-efficiency of nursing. Nevertheless, others question the adequacy of the research basis of nursing in relation to cost (Maynard 1994).

The white paper (DoH 1997) envisages a National Institute of Clinical Effectiveness, with a remit to disseminate cost-effective practice, combined with a national schedule of reference costs, in which costs relating to performance between trusts will be assessed. These developments will reinforce concern about cost which is likely to emerge as the single most important issue for nurses of the future, determining the nature of the relationship between professional nurses and managers and the process of management (Wells 1996).

Conclusion

Nursing draws its membership from a wide range of the population and so it is not surprising that it reflects societal preoccupations and social progress (Bevis 1983). Since the 1960s UK society has become dominated increasingly by economic principles encapsulated in a rational managerialism. Nursing's vulnerability in terms of the sheer size and cost of its workforce, coupled with its traditional deference to perceived authority, helps explain why management changes have impacted on nursing perhaps more than on any other clinical group. The career structure of nurses now stresses function and does not necessarily require a clinical nursing qualification for a clinical management post, though in practice those employed tend to have one. Ends through cost-effective means is confirmed by the 1997 white paper (DoH 1997) as a primary concern for health care managers. In future nurses will be employed only if they can meet this criterion. This has profound implications not only for what nurses actually do but for the whole conception of what we mean when we ask 'what is a nurse?'. The increased emphasis on resource management, devolved budgeting, cost-effective interventions, clinical governance and an increased role in commissioning will change the identity and the focus of work for nurses who take on those responsibilities. It is a management agenda that will dictate the parameters of clinical work and change the language of nursing, as management concepts of cost efficiency, corporate identity and accountability are internalised.

References

Abel-Smith, B. (1964) *The Hospitals 1800–1948: A Study in Social Administration.* Heinemann, London.

Ackroyd, S. (1995) Nurses, management and morale: a diagnosis of decline in the NHS hospital service. In: *Interprofessional Relations in Health Care*, (eds K. Soothill, L. Mackay & C. Webb), pp. 222–38. Edward Arnold, London.

Audit Commission (1991) *The Virtue of Patients: Making the Best Use of Ward Nursing Resources.* HMSO, London.

Baly, M. (1986) *Florence Nightingale and the Nursing Legacy.* Croom Helm, London.

Baly, M. (1995) *Nursing and Social Change*. Routledge, London.

Beecher, C. & Couchey, C. (1997) Had a nice day? *Health Service Journal*, **107**(5567) 28–9.

Benner, P. (1984) *From Novice to Expert*. Addison-Wesley, Menlo Park, California.

Bevis, E.O. (1983) *Curriculum Building in Nursing – A Process*, (3rd edn). C.V. Mosby, St Louis.

Burns, D. (1998) Trouble Zones? *Health Service Journal*, 28 February, p. 9.

Carpenter, M. (1980) *All for One*. Confederation of Health Service Employees, Banstead.

Carr, A.J. (1978) The work of the nursing officer. *Nursing Times*, **74**(23), 89–92.

Carr-Hill, R. Dixon, J. & Gibbs, I. (1992) *Skill Mix and Effectiveness of Nursing Care*. Centre for Health Economics, University of York.

Checkland, P. & Scholes, J. (1992) *Soft Systems Methodology in Action*. John Wiley & Sons, Chichester.

Clark, J. (1995) Nurses as managers. In: Nursing And Social Change, (ed. M.E. Baly), 3rd edn, pp. 277–94. Routledge, London.

Clay, T. (1987) *Nurses, Power and Politics*. Heinemann Nursing, London.

Connechen, J. (1991) Research in nursing management. In: *The Research Process in Nursing* (ed. D. Cormack), (2nd edn). Blackwell Science, Oxford.

Cowie, V. (1995) Nursing, economic change and industrial relations. In: *Nursing And Social Change*, (ed. M.E. Baly), pp. 337–51. (3rd edn), Routledge, London.

Cowpe, J. (1995) Managing within the organisation. In: *The Clinician's Management Handbook*, (eds D. Hansell & B. Salter). W.B. Saunders Co Ltd, London.

Dawson, S., Winstanley, D., Mole, V. & Sherval, J. (1996) *Managing in the NHS: A Study of Senior Executives*. The Management School Imperial College, London.

Dennis, T. (1997) Getting the measure of the NHS. *Health Service Journal*, **107**(5560), 18.

Department of State and Official Bodies, Ministry of Health, National Health Service, National Nursing Staff Committee (1968) *A Report by the National Staff Committee on Management Development of Senior Nursing Staff in the Hospital Service*. HMSO, London.

DHSS (Department of Health and Social Security) (1969) *Report of the Working Party on Management Structure in the local authority nursing service (Mayston Report)*. HMSO, London.

DHSS (Department of Health and Social Security) (1972) *Report of the Committee on Nursing (Briggs Committee)*. HMSO, London.

DHSS (Department of Health and Social Security) (1983) *National Health Service Management Inquiry*. HMSO, London.

DoH (Department of Health) (1989a) *Working for Patients*. HMSO, London.

DoH (Department of Health) (1989b) *A Strategy for Nursing*. HMSO, London.

DoH (Department of Health) (1991) *The Patient's Charter*. HMSO, London.

DoH (Department of Health) (1997) *The New NHS: modern–dependable*. (White paper, Cmnd 3807). The Stationery Office, London.

DoH (Department of Health) (1998) *Press Release – Today Marks Radical New Direction for NHS – Frank Dobson*. 1 April, 98–124.

Drucker, P.F. (1993) *The Practice of Management*. Butterworth Heinemann, Oxford.

Duffield, C.M. & Lumby, J. (1994) Context and culture – the influence on role transition for first-line nurse managers. *International Journal of Nursing Studies*, **31**(6), 555–60.

Eby, M. (1994) Competing values. In: *Ethics – Conflicts of Interests*, (ed. V. Tschudin). Scutari Press, London.

Enthoven, A. (1985) *Reflections on the Management of the National Health Service.* Nuffield Provincial Hospitals Trust, London.

Evans, A. (1993) Accountability: a core concept for primary nursing. *Journal of Clinical Nursing,* 2, 231–4.

Fowler, J. (1984) Learning to be a ward sister. *Nurse Education Today,* 5(6), 231–6.

Fox, N. (1992) *The Social Meaning of Surgery.* The Open University, Milton Keynes.

Gabe, J., Kelleher, D. & Williams, G. (eds) (1994) *Challenging Medicine.* Routledge, London.

Gavin, J.N. (1995) The politics of nursing: a case study – clinical grading. *Journal of Advanced Nursing,* 22, 379–85.

du Gay, P. (1996) Making up managers: enterprise and the ethos of bureaucracy. In: *The Politics of Management Knowledge,* (eds S.R. Clegg & G. Palmer), pp. 19–35. Sage, London.

GNC (1982) *Training syllabus, Register of nurses, Mental Nursing.* General Nursing Council for England & Wales, London.

Gray, A. & Jenkins, B. (1995) Public management and the NHS. In: *Managing Health Care Challenges for the 1990s* (eds J.J. Glynn & D.A. Perkins) pp. 4–32. W.B. Saunders, London.

Hadley, R. & Clough, R. (1996) *Care in Chaos – Frustration and Challenge in Community Care.* Cassell, London.

Ham, C. (1992) *Health Policy in Britain,* (3rd edn). Macmillan, Hong Kong.

Hancock, C. (1994) Ignore us at your peril. *Health Service Journal,* 104(5408), 21.

Hancock, C. (1996) With the benefit of foresight. *Health Service Journal,* 106(5509) 23.

Hancock, C. (1997) Careless cutting remarks. *Health Service Journal,* 106(5485), 19.

Harrison, S., Hunter, D.J. Marnoch, G. & Pollitt, C. (1992) *Just Managing: Power and Culture in the National Health Service.* Macmillan, London.

Harrison, S. & Pollitt, C. (1994) *Controlling Health Professionals: The Future of Work and Organization in the NHS.* Open University Press, Milton Keynes.

Haywood, S.C. (1968) The unwilling managers. *British Hospital Journal and Social Service Review,* **LXXVIII**(4061), 297–8.

Healthcare 2000 (1995) *UK Health and Healthcare Services Challenges and Policy Options.* University of Manchester, Manchester.

Hunter, D.J. (1993) To market! To market! A new dawn for community care? *Health and Social Care in the Community,* 1, 3–10.

Hunter, D.J. (1996) Give merit where it's due. *Health Service Journal,* 106(5495), 21.

Johnson, S., Brooks, L., Sutherby, K., Thornicroft, G., Johnson, C. & Loftus, L. (1997) Sending in the Paras. *Health Service Journal,* 107(5570), 30–31.

Jowett, S. (1996) *Every nurse's business – the role of marketing on service.* King's Fund, London.

Keen, J. & Malby, R. (1992) Nursing power and practice in the United Kingdom National Health Service. *Journal of Advanced Nursing,* 17, 863–70.

Kenrick, M. & Luker, K. (1996) An exploration of the influence of managerial factors on research utilisation in district nursing practice. *Journal of Advanced Nursing,* 23, 697–704.

La Monica, E. (1990) *Management in Health Care: A Theoretical and Experiential Approach.* Macmillan, London.

Lathlean, J. & Farnish, S. (1984) *The Ward Sister Training Project: an evaluation of a training scheme for ward sisters.* Nurse Education Research Unit, Dept. of Nursing Studies, Chelsea College, University of London.

Leathard, A. (1990) *Health Care Provision Past Present and Future.* Chapman and Hall, London.

Levitt, R. & Wall, A. (1989) *The Reorganised National Health Service*, (3rd edn). Chapman and Hall, London.

Lipsky, M. (1980) *Street Level Bureaucracy*. Plenum Press, New York.

Martin, J. & Siehl, C. (1983) Organizational culture and counterculture: an uneasy symbiosis. *Organizational Dynamics*, Autumn, 52–64.

Matthews, A. & Whelan, J. (1995) *In Charge of the Ward*, (3rd edn). Blackwell Science, Oxford.

Maynard, A. (1994) Who is managing nurses? *Health Service Journal*, **104**(5411), 19.

Maynard, A. (1997a) School for scandal. *Health Service Journal*, **107**(5567), 20.

Maynard, A. (1997b) Time to send on the subs. *Health Service Journal*, **107**(5537), 20.

Maynard, A. (1998) Happy days are here again. *Health Service Journal*, 29 January, p. 20.

McKee, I. & Laing, W. (1993) *Rationing Medicine*. Association of the British Pharmaceutical Industry, London.

McSweeney, P. (1991) The collapse of the conventional career. *Nursing Times*, **87**(31), 26–8.

MHSHHD (Ministry of Health, Scottish Home and Health Department) (1966) *Report of the Committee on Senior Nursing Staff Structure* (chaired by Salmon). HMSO, London.

O'Kelly, R. (1989) *Pricing the NHS: A Resource Management Initiative*. The Greater London Association of Community Health Councils, London.

Oni, O. (1997) Managers: who needs them? *Health Service Journal*, **107**(5539), 20.

Onyett, S., Pillinger, T. & Muijen, M. (1996) Job satisfaction and burn out among members of community mental health teams. *Journal of Mental Health*, **6**(1), 55–66.

Oroviogoicoechea, C. (1996) The clinical nurse manager: a literature review. *Journal of Advanced Nursing*, 24, 1273–80.

Owens, P. & Glennerster, H. (1987) Aiming for the Top. *Nursing Times*, 83, 35–7.

Owens, P. & Glennerster, H. (1990) *Nursing in Conflict*. Macmillan, London.

Paton, C. (1996) *Health Policy and Management: The Healthcare Agenda in a British Political Context*. Chapman Hall, London.

Pembrey, S. (1978) *The role of the ward sister in the management of nursing – a study of the organisation of nursing on an individualised patient basis*. PhD thesis, University of Edinburgh.

Porter, S. (1992) The poverty of professionalisation: a critical analysis of strategies for the occupational advancement of nursing. *Journal of Advanced Nursing*, 17, 720–26.

Rawlins, C. (1992) *Introduction to Management*. Harper Collins, New York.

RCN Management Association (1989) *Standards of Care for Management in Nursing*. Royal College of Nursing, London.

Redfern, S. (1981) *Hospital Sisters: their job satisfaction and occupational stability*. Royal College of Nursing, London.

Reed, M. (1989) *The Sociology of Management*. Harvester Wheatsheaf, New York.

Roberts, C. (1996) The Proof of the pudding. *Health Service Journal*, **106**(5494), 27.

Roberts, J.A. (1989) From myths to markets. *Health and Policy Planning*, **4**(1), 62–71.

Royal College of Surgeons (1998) *The Primary Health Care Team*. RCGP Information Sheet No 21. Royal College of General Practitioners Information Services web site http://www.rcgp.org.uk/informat/publicat/rcf0021.htm

Salter, B. & Snee, N. (1997) Power dressing. *Health Service Journal*, **107**(5540), 30–31.

Savage, S.P. & Robins, L. (eds) (1990) *Public Policy under Thatcher*. Macmillan, London.

Schurr, M. (1968) *Leadership and the Nurse: An Introduction to the Principles of Management*. The English Universities Press, London.

Small, N. (1989) *Politics and Planning in the National Health Service*. Open University Press, Milton Keynes.

Strong, P. & Robinson, J. (1990) *The NHS Under New Management*. Open University Press, Milton Keynes.

Suomin, T., Kovasin, M. & Ketola, O. (1997) Nursing culture – some viewpoints. *Journal of Advanced Nursing*, 25, 186–90.

Taylor, F.W. (1911) *The Principles of Scientific Management*. Harper Row, New York.

UKCC (1986) *Project 2000: A New Preparation for Practice*. UKCC, London.

Wells, J.S.G. (1994) Analysis of health rationing policies in the NHS. *British Journal of Nursing*, 3(4), 188–91.

Wells, J.S.G. (1995a) Health care rationing: nursing perspectives. *Journal of Advanced Nursing*, 22, 738–44.

Wells, J.S.G. (1995b) Discontent without focus? An analysis of nurse management activity on a psychiatric in-patient facility using a 'soft systems' approach. *Journal of Advanced Nursing*, 21, 214–21.

Wells, J.S.G. (1996) The public/professional interface with priority setting in the NHS. *Journal of Health and Social Care in the Community*, 5, 2.

White, R. (1985) *The Effects of the NHS on the Nursing Profession 1948–61*. King's Fund, London.

Wiggins, L. (1997) The conflict between 'new nursing' and 'scientific management' as perceived by surgical nurses. *Journal of Advanced Nursing*, 25, 1116–22.

Wilkinson, M.J. (1995) Love is not a marketable commodity: new public management in the British National Health Service. *Journal of Advanced Nursing*, 21, 980–87.

Wilson-Barnett, J. (1973) The work of the unit nursing officer. *Nursing Times Occasional Papers*, **69**(24), 97–9; **69**(25), 101–103.

Wilson-Barnett, J. (1988) Nursing values: exploring the clichés. *Journal of Advanced Nursing*, 13, 790–96.

Wilson-Barnett, J. & Beech, S. (1995) Evaluating the Clinical Nurse Specialist. A review. *International Journal of Nursing Studies*, **31**(6), 561–72.

Witz, A. (1994) The challenge of nursing. In: *Challenging Medicine*, (eds J. Gabe, D. Kelleher & G. Williams), pp. 23–45. Routledge, London.

Wolin, S.S. (1961) *Politics and Vision: Continuity and Innovation in Western Political Thought*. Oxford University Press, Oxford.

Yassin, T. (1996) Ward sisters' views of the effects of NHS changes. *Nursing Times*, **92**(20) 32–3.

5 Nursing Skill: Potential or Dilution?

Margaret Edwards

Fears that nursing would be diminished as a therapeutic endeavour if a hands-on role were to be relinquished are often voiced. Such fears are fuelled by recommendations that support workers could perform many of the tasks currently thought to be the domain of nursing and the view that numbers of these workers should double in the early years following the millennium (Health Services Management Unit 1996). Others, however, have argued (DHSS 1972, Salvage 1988) that unqualified assistants have always provided hands-on care and are the backbone of the health service.

Historically, the demand for nursing has always outstripped the supply of nurses (Abel-Smith 1960). Demographic pressures in the form of an ageing population with high levels of disability and chronic illness, together with a shortfall in the number of candidates available for nurse training make it unlikely that basic nursing care will ever be delivered exclusively by qualified staff. Lisbeth Hockey (1978) made this point as long ago as the late 1970s before the advent of Project 2000 (UKCC 1986) and the removal of students from the workforce. The question of how nursing is going to deal with a growing army of unqualified staff within its workforce has acquired some urgency.

This chapter examines the position of unqualified assistants within nursing and evaluates the effects of distancing the registered nurse from the 'bedside'. Much of the chapter is concerned with a historical overview of nursing and the unqualified worker. This is because a review of the past has much to offer in dispelling some mythologies of nursing and the often irrational fears that have grown up around the unqualified worker. Much of the discussion takes place against the backdrop of the increasing demands for health care and a restructured health service brought into line with current managerial thinking in its emphasis on flexibility, efficiency and cost-effectiveness. The lessons of history suggest a way forward that includes embracing the unqualified worker as well as establishing a role for nursing that is both in line with its therapeutic commitment and its professional aspirations within a managerial age.

Mythologies of nursing

Anxieties arising from the prospect of unqualified support workers delivering direct care could be said to stem from a view of nursing that is embedded in the nineteenth century stereotype of the Nightingale nurse, stationed by the bedside. The powerful image of the lady and the lamp exists in the collective psyche of both the public and the profession, but as the Briggs Report (DHSS 1972) pointed out, these images may be different from reality. Most paid caring in the nineteenth and well into the twentieth century was in fact carried out by untrained 'handywomen' (Dingwall *et al.* 1988). Dingwall *et al.* have disputed the portrayal of Florence Nightingale in the Crimea as the bedside nurse, remarking that most of the care was given, as it always had been, by ward orderlies and soldiers' wives. The success of Florence Nightingale and her companions at Scutari appears to have lain in their organisational skills in the face of military incompetence. However, the portrayal of this selfless upper-class lady 'up to her neck in muck and bullets' captured the imagination of the time. It is an image that has existed ever since. Curiously, history largely ignored the role of Mrs Seacole, the Creole nurse whose contribution to the front line care of soldiers in the Crimea from all accounts rivalled if not surpassed that of Florence Nightingale (Alexander & Dewjee 1984). Mrs Seacole, an ordinary woman from the West Indies, did not capture the nineteenth century imagination!

Further mythologies

The second half of the nineteenth century witnessed the growth of professional nursing. Training became available in foundations such as the Nightingale School. Interestingly though, in the Nightingale School basic bedside care, in terms of washing and feeding, was not given by the probationer nurses but rather by 'under nurses' who also carried out manual household chores. Abel-Smith (1960) suggested that the Nightingale School was in practice more important as a training school for matrons than as a training school for nurses. Training schools such as those at St Thomas' Hospital retained all the features of the Victorian household where servants had traditionally cared for the sick.

In the community the early district nursing schemes in Liverpool depended heavily on supervision of the 'nurses' by lady superintendents. This division of labour is also evident in the early health visiting schemes as 'mission women' recruited from the handywomen class were not trusted to work on their own. They were again supervised by a lady volunteer (Dingwall *et al.* 1988). The notion of the trained nurse as supervisor recurs throughout the history of the profession and will be revisited later in this chapter with respect to current developments in nursing.

The need for professional nurses

If Dickensian accounts of the care afforded to sick inmates of the workhouse are to be believed, a need for proper supervision of the 'handywomen nurses' was undoubtedly needed. The portrayal of the handywoman in literature is typified by the unwholesome character Sarah Gamp. However Abel-Smith (1960) has reminded us that reformers were likely to embellish their case. He has also pointed to evidence from the 1866 Lancet Sanitary Commission that care given by pauper nurses was not uniformly bad. Nolan (1993) in his history of mental health nursing has mentioned the description of exemplary care given by untrained assistants to the terminally ill in the Colney Hatch asylum in 1859.

Nonetheless, Florence Nightingale's perceived success in the Crimea, the need for close observation of patients arising from advances in medicine and the growth of philanthropic and religious movements all fuelled the demand for better nursing. In theory the establishment of training schools in many of the voluntary hospitals, and the provision for training in selected poor law institutions under the Metropolitan Poor Act 1867 (section 29), should have heralded the demise of the pauper nurse and the handywoman. In practice the numbers of untrained nurses grew exponentially. The reasons for their continued survival are twofold. First, as has already been mentioned, demand for nursing care outstripped supply. Secondly, the 'respectable' lady probationers were unlikely to seek employment in the poor law institutions and even those who had been recruited for training in the poor law asylums were keen to leave to seek better employment elsewhere (Abel-Smith 1960).

The poor law institutions catered for the chronically sick and incurable, while nursing in the voluntary hospitals provided more opportunity for the exercise of skills. A cachet of respectability was attached to working within a voluntary hospital and the argument could therefore be upheld that nursing was a suitable profession for middle class women. The same argument could not be made for nursing the chronic sick within the poor law institutions where matrons were few and far between and nurses would have been in the employ of workhouse masters who were their social inferiors. Nevertheless, the workhouse infirmaries had to be staffed and this was achieved by employing ever larger numbers of untrained nurses (Abel-Smith 1960).

The numbers of untrained staff in all areas of nursing increased particularly during World War I. The influx of the Voluntary Aid Detachment (VAD) (Roberts 1996) sharpened the argument within the profession for a register so that nursing could retain its aspirations as a suitable career for educated women. The effects of registration were in fact to concentrate trained nursing in the voluntary hospitals and on the district (Abel-Smith 1960). Unqualified nurses continued to plug the gap, staffing the mushrooming number of nursing homes and, as Abel-Smith (1960) acknowledged, while the care of the acutely sick was undoubtedly improved, the fate of the chronic sick may have been made worse. The dependence on untrained nursing labour has certainly been an enduring feature of elderly care (Davies 1992).

The division of labour in health care

It was in the voluntary hospitals that the need for the more educated type of nurse was most keenly felt. Medical advances made careful observation vital. Experienced and skilled nursing made delegation and consequent medical consultant status possible (Garmarnikow 1991). It has been pointed out that:

'one of the fundamental processes of the division of labour in health care is the making of innovations by doctors which once routinised are then delegated to nurses or other paramedical staff.'

(Dingwall *et al.* 1988, p. 164)

Resistance to this process, very much evident today in the debate over the extended role of the nurse and substitutions of role (Hunt & Wainwright 1994), does not take into account the historical fact that nursing tasks such as dressing wounds and urine testing were in the Victorian hospital the exclusive domain of the physician or physician's assistant. These tasks are now so much part of nursing routine that they are jealously guarded, as they once were by medical staff (Garmarnikow 1991), and often auxiliary staff are not trusted to perform them (Rye 1978, Mersey RHA 1989). Yet according to Dingwall *et al.* (1988), divisions of labour are not static but rather like cities take on new forms to adapt to changing social pressures. In the past, physiotherapy constituted just such a development and it may be that in the nursing support worker a new division of labour is evolving in response to social pressures.

Medicine, by leaving the bedside, gained higher status (Garmanikow 1991). In discussing professionalisation, Ramprogus (1995) outlines the process whereby as professionals increase their repertoire of knowledge and skills, areas of work are generated which are seen as menial and more appropriate to be carried out by lower level workers. Thus doctors abandoned dressing wounds and testing urine to nurses, while they engaged in higher level practice based on theoretical forms of knowledge. Ramprogus (1995) has argued that 'ditching the dirty work' is a necessary component in the professionalising process. By establishing a register in 1919, nursing achieved what is known as social closure, another important feature of professionalisation. Weber, cited in Murphy (1988), described social closure as the process by which social collectives seek to maximise rewards by restricting access to resources and opportunities to a limited circle of eligibles. Ramprogus (1995) again contends that in achieving social closure nursing, like other professions, had to undergo internal divisions, resulting in the development of subgroups. The eventual creation of the second level or enrolled nurse after the setting up of the register is an example of just such a division. The (literally) 'dirty work' in nursing has largely been the domain of the enrolled nurse and the nursing auxiliary.

Nursing within a social and political context

Dingwall *et al.* (1988) have suggested that divisions of labour arise because of social pressures. Indeed it would seem unlikely that professions could arise and achieve social closure simply through the volition of their prospective members alone. A review of the social, economic and political history of the nineteenth and twentieth centuries provides an explanation as to why nursing was able to achieve closure through the setting up and maintenance of a register. Political, social and economic factors also explain the manner in which nursing has been organised (Lister 1997). Organisation of work within a profession might seem to be a question for that profession alone but is in fact governed by prevailing ideology and must be seen within that context.

Prior to the 1970s, models of nursing existed which revolved around task allocation. These reflected theories of scientific management that were being implemented in the industrial world (McKeown 1995). Henry Ford developed the production line, where, in the name of efficiency, specific tasks were assigned to individuals. This type of factory production became the model for other types of work and Lister (1997) has compared the task allocation system of nursing to Ford's production line. According to Lister (1997) the essential task of the nurse was to complete allocated routines rather than to be concerned with the 'whole patient'. This way of working resembled that of the car factory worker who was concerned only with the specific task and not with the construction of the 'whole car'. This system of working has been referred to as 'Fordism' (McKeown 1995). The organisation of nursing work shadowed political and industrial structures.

Redefining nursing

Nursing remained enmeshed in social processes even when it attempted from the 1960s onwards to define itself as a unique activity separate from medicine. Lister (1997 p. 41) describes the humanistic trends in nursing as having been 'inescapably shaped by the Enlightenment discourse of the primacy of the individual'. Virginia Henderson's classic definition of the function of the nurse marked a watershed in the thinking of nursing. Her definition established the nurse's function as being concerned with the individual at the interpersonal level (Lister 1997). With this individualised focus the ideological basis of nursing shifted from task allocation and subservience to a medical model towards holistic, patient-centred care. Primary nursing, which involved allocating 24 hour responsibility for each patient's care to a registered nurse, became a preferred method of work organisation (Ramprogus 1995). This is not to say, however, that it became the *actual* method of work organisation as recent research has reported that task allocation is alive and well, particularly in elderly care (Koch & Webb 1996).

It could not be entirely coincidental that in the same period that Virginia Henderson was framing her famous definition of nursing, the hippy movement with its focus on love and the freedom of the individual was born in the USA. The humanistic zeitgeist of the late 1960s and 1970s was also visible in the work of psychologists and educational theorists of the period. In 1969 Rogers published his influential theory of personal growth which stressed the importance of the self and self-concept (Rogers 1969). Within the NHS consensus management was the order of the day.

The ideological shift in nursing from a subservience model (whether to the bureaucracy or to medicine) to a professional model wherein the nurse became, in Virginia Henderson's words, the 'initiator' and 'master' of the care she delivered, involved a reappraisal of the nature of that care (Henderson 1966, p. 15). Rye (1978) has described the feeling within nursing that basic care – the real stuff of nursing – had been usurped and needed to be reclaimed for registered nurses, and that it had to be invested with new meaning which put it beyond the capabilities of all but the registered nurse. This feeling found expression in the concept of primary nursing with its emphasis on interpersonal relationships and therapeutic care. It has been suggested that therapeutic care occurs when nurses understand their primary caring function and have a positive approach to patients' health (Kitson 1991).

It is curious that the profession should believe that basic care had to be reclaimed for registered nurses since there is little evidence historically that outside specialist units such care was ever delivered exclusively by registered nurses. Indeed it could be argued that any usurping that has taken place has been on the part of trained nurses hijacking that care that was traditionally undertaken by the handywoman class! Studies of nursing activity in units providing care for elderly people persistently reveal that the majority of direct care is and has been provided by nursing auxiliaries (Adams & McIllwraith 1963, Wells 1980, Phillips 1988, Davies 1992).

It seems easy for those whom Thomas (1992) refers to as the professionalisers or proselytisers to forget that prior to Project 2000 (UKCC 1986), learners made up a large section of the nursing workforce. It is possible that in looking back to a golden age in which the trained nurse reigned supreme, the profession has confused the presence of the registered nurse with that of the learner. However those who argue for an all qualified workforce do so on the basis of achieving better outcomes for their patients (Pearson 1988, MacMahon 1989). Koch and Webb's (1996) study of an elderly care hospital setting found that patients' wishes were ignored in favour of 'routine practice' when care was given by untrained auxiliaries and enrolled nurses. The professionalisers argue that better quality care results when trained nurses deliver basic care. They argue that not only is quality enhanced but that registered nurses are also more cost effective and cost efficient (Pearson 1988, MacMahon 1989).

Qualified versus unqualified staff

Leaders of the profession point to studies emanating from the USA, and in the UK, such as the study by Carr-Hill *et al.* (1992) to demonstrate that qualified staff are both cost-effective and cost efficient (Hancock quoted in Seymour 1992). McKenna (1995) in a review of studies relating to skill mix has noted that transatlantic studies are not easily translatable. In testing out assumptions about skill mix, McKenna came to the conclusion that a sufficient number of studies are available which can be used to support the retention of a large number of registered nurses, although few demonstrate the necessary rigour for lobbying purposes. The problem however with studies such as the much quoted Carr-Hill *et al.* (1992) study is that the researchers make comparisons between nurses who have undergone formal education and training and staff for whom training is likely to have been sparse if not non-existent. A more valid approach would be to compare qualified (trained staff) with unqualified but trained staff.

Further Carr-Hill *et al.*'s study is problematic on other counts. The authors claim their convenience sample of seven hospitals was representative. However, they selected their subjects for observation purposively even though randomisation could have been used and indeed would have been desirable since one of the instruments used, Qualpacs (Wandelt & Ager 1974), requires randomisation of patients for observation. The researchers chose to use high dependency patients in the hope of securing a high number of observations. In selecting these patients the study was immediately likely to disadvantage untrained staff as many of the tasks under consideration were not those traditionally undertaken by auxiliaries, e.g. monitoring the rate of intravenous infusions and arranging discharge.

Despite this, Carr Hill *et al.*'s study is frequently held up as proof of the advantages of a trained nursing workforce. However, there is evidence to show that where qualified staff only are used, effectiveness may suffer. Ahmed and Kitson (1993) noted that in community hospital units where primary nurses were the principal care-givers, regardless of whether the patient constantly needed qualified input, continuity and consistency in the quality of care could not be maintained in the absence of the primary nurse. In these units auxiliaries were found to have a very small input towards direct patient care. Reluctance on the part of a large section of the profession to recognise the contribution of the nursing support worker or to offer a coherent programme of training is by no means new. By the early 1970s the urgent need for training had been recognised (DHSS 1972).

The training of unqualified staff

The Committee on Nursing (Briggs Report) (DHSS 1972), recognising the dependence of the nursing and midwifery system on nursing auxiliaries and assistants, believed the education of 'nursing aides' to be a matter of considerable urgency. The Committee commented on the fragmentary nature of education for unqualified staff and the lack of any general regulation of provision for training. The survey carried out for the Committee on Nursing found that in over 50% of hospitals no training at all, induction or later instruction, was offered to nursing aides. Half the auxiliaries in the representative sample reported that they had received no training at all. The Committee's recommendations for in-service training seem to have been largely ignored.

Other surveys of training provision for untrained staff consistently demonstrate a lack of training for unqualified staff (Hardie 1978, Thomas

1992). Hardie (1978) in a national study of auxiliary usage (response rate 88.6% of all districts) found that 70% of districts offered orientation days and/or in-service training. Hardie found, however, that the time devoted to training was only partially quantifiable. In approximately one third of the 30 pilot interviews carried out with auxiliaries, it was revealed that even though the hospitals concerned did offer some instruction on a formal basis, the individual interviewed had not received the training for one reason or another. In only 31% of the districts was the instruction offered under the auspices of the nurse education system.

More recently Thomas (1992) in her thesis comparing the work of registered nurses and nursing auxiliaries in primary, team and functional nursing wards found that her sample of auxiliaries suffered from the same lack of training. In a study examining the role of the support worker in the health care team, Robinson *et al.* (1989) described how, despite considerable length of employment, systematic attention to training had not apparently been paid to any of the traditional support worker roles. While and Barriball (1994) had similar findings. Carr-Hill *et al.* (1992), in their study of nursing skill mix, found that, apart from wards on which primary nursing was practised, most staff received very little training and unqualified staff the least of all. This lack of training has implications for the quality of care given to patients but also raises doubts about the validity of those skill mix studies that attempt to compare the quality and effectiveness of qualified versus unqualified nurses.

Historically the lack of training for unqualified staff reflects the profession's general antipathy towards the nursing assistant. Dickson and Cole (1987) have claimed that 'rather like sex and death, nursing assistants are essential, but that does not make them suitable topics for polite conversation' (Dickson & Cole 1987, p. 24). The profession has longed for the day when only the qualified would reign. Some look forward to an all graduate profession (Day 1994). Paradoxically, the major change in nurse education of recent years, the introduction of Project 2000 (UKCC 1986), required the replacement of the student workforce with health care assistants. The fact that the UKCC had to concede to this new division of labour illustrates perhaps just how much bedside nursing has been carried out by students. There has, however, to date been sparse and sporadic enthusiasm for nursing involvement in the training of this new breed of support worker. The title 'health care assistant' studiously avoids the use of the word nurse or nursing and again suggests the profession's reluctance to embrace the new worker as part of the nursing team. Yet health care assistants are here to stay and are more than likely to increase. The reasons for this are both demographic and political.

Demographic considerations

It has been noted already that the greater part of the twentieth century has been marked by the demand for nursing care exceeding supply. Nurse shortages are again on the agenda with reports of trusts having to provide

material enticements to recruit staff (Leifer 1996). Difficulties in recruitment vary but a shortfall of 12 to 14% has been found in some areas
(Boulton 1996). Without 'an independent, robust systematic and independent review of nurse staffing levels' (Seccombe 1996, p. 25), it is difficult to
disentangle what has been reported as 'a little local difficulty' in recruitment from any wider trend. According to Buchan (1997) the NHS reforms
resulting from the NHS and Community Care Act 1990, have made
detailed, standardised aggregation of local workforce data more difficult.

In the past, responses to the problem were not those most palatable to the
profession, that is the creation of a second level nurse in 1943 (Abel-Smith
1960) and the reduction of the educational entry requirements. It is
estimated that 50% of the 18 year old population with 5 GCSE grade Cs or
above or with 2 A-levels will need to be recruited in order to meet the
requirements of the NHS qualified health-care practitioners (Townsend
1989). The traditional recruitment pattern to nursing, together with known
demographic trends, is already producing a shortfall of entrants to nursing
which will continue well into the next century (DHSS 1987, Waite 1989).
Price Waterhouse, on behalf of the UKCC, have estimated that the cumu-
lative shortfall of entrants by the year 2004 will be in the region of 10 000
(DHSS 1987). In the decade between 1984 and 1994 the number of student
nurses halved (Buchan 1997).

An increasingly competitive employment market and doubts as to the
desirability of the NHS as an employer have also been cited as possible
reasons for this trend (Townsend 1989). It will be difficult for nursing to
compete with other employers, for instance financial institutions in the
private sector who already provide child-care facilities at the workplace
(Waite 1989), without a radical change in recruitment and retention policies
which make it easier for women to combine family and career responsibilities. Even if sufficient numbers of potential candidates were to be
available it is not every person who is equipped psychologically and
emotionally to be a nurse (Abel-Smith 1960), a point illustrated by the
historically high level of attrition from nurse training (MoH 1939).

Meeting the needs of those with chronic illness

This ongoing problem with recruitment and retention in nursing exists
against the backdrop of an increase in the numbers of the 'old' elderly
(Central Statistical Office 1996). Some people hold optimistic views about
the health status of this population, believing that improved standards of
living will contribute to a compression of morbidity, that is disabling illness
will feature only for a short period prior to death (Fries 1980, 1996, Manton
1982). There is, though, an opposing view which sees this generation as
representing the failures of medical success (Gruenberg 1977, Moody 1995),
that is elderly people for whom death has been postponed by medical
advances but who consequently live for long periods with high levels of
chronic disease and reduced quality of life, and make increasing demands

on health and social services. There is some evidence in support of this view (Bowling *et al.* 1993).

The highest admission rates from heart failure in a London hospital are among those 75 years of age and over and are most marked in the over 85s (Majeed 1993). North American studies suggest that as many as one third of recurrent hospitalisations could be prevented (Hawthorne & Hickson 1993). Studies do not distinguish between progression of the disease and lack of compliance but Hawthorne and Hickson (1993) have suggested that inadequate symptom management may be the precipitating factor in many hospitalisations. Symptoms include weight gain, oedema and dyspnoea (Masiello Millar 1994). Close monitoring of both the signs and symptoms of congestive heart failure is held to be essential to long-term follow-up once the diagnosis of congestive heart failure is established (Masiello Millar 1994). In the UK, with increasing numbers of 'old' elderly living on their own (Central Statistical Office 1996) the question of who will be monitoring for acute-on-chronic exacerbations of diseases such as congestive heart failure or chronic obstructive airways disease needs to be explored.

The Value for Money Unit's study of district nursing skill mix (NHSME 1992), although criticised for its task orientated approach (Cowley 1993), does provide information on the nature and frequency of diagnostic tasks such as weighing and blood pressure monitoring based on a total of 5721 visits by all grades of district nursing staff across three community trusts. Blood pressure measurement took place on 0.07% visits and weighing on 0.01%. None of these tasks were undertaken by auxiliary staff. If the results of the Value for Money study in terms of monitoring of patient condition can be generalised it seems unlikely that the monitoring needs of an increasing chronically sick population can be met within existing resources or methods of working. Pearson and Wistow (1995) have noted that long term care has been associated historically with inappropriate institutional arrangements and inadequate community care provision.

There is evidence in the literature, and particularly in the literature concerned with lay carers (Nolan & Grant 1989; Pearson & Wistow 1995), that the district nursing service has never adequately succeeded in meeting the needs of all the old and sick in the community (Skeet & Crout 1977; Heslop & Bagnell 1988). Heslop and Bagnell (1988) in their intervention study of patients with disabling chest disease (*n* = 75) found that most of the elderly and disabled participants were not being visited by a district nurse or health visitor. In their survey of 250 patients Skeet & Crout (1977) found that 22% of long stay patients and 15% of short stay patients needed help with basic care such as washing and dressing when they reached home and were not receiving it. Carers of old people who were sick needed information on pressure area care, the management of constipation and incontinence and how to change a soiled drawsheet. Skeet (1978) concluded that the members of the primary health care team, as it was then composed, could not give the help as often as it was required and that a skill mix was needed which included teaching preparation for an auxiliary, providing support for the nurse responsible for overall care.

Skill mix

Buchan (1997) has warned that while nursing shortages may provide leverage for trade unions in the pay arena, they are also likely to refocus attention on new working patterns and skill mix. Cost containment of health care is a national and international goal (ICN 1993) and nursing accounts for a large proportion of the NHS wage bill. Hockey (1978) argued in the 1970s that any public service which is not self-limiting must find ways to control expenditure and that nursing is an economic activity, a fact that has been largely ignored by the profession until recently. As demand for health care continues to grow, purchasers are increasingly likely to challenge staff costs of provider units (Health Services Management Unit 1996).

Indeed nursing staff establishments have been the focus of much recent scrutiny (Audit Commission 1991, NHSME 1992). The Audit Commission (1991) found considerable variations in ratios of qualified to unqualified staff. The proportion of qualified staff was found to vary from 49% to 72% in acute general hospital wards. Variations were found between similar trusts and between similar services within trusts. In the community the number of G and H grade nurses as a proportion of the nursing team was also found to vary considerably (NHSME 1992); it seems likely that nursing establishments in the community have been historically determined rather than planned in relation to workload (Audit Commission 1992). The National Health Service Management Executive Value for Money Unit (VFMU) (NHSME 1992) contended that 'the appropriate skill mix should be that which is based on an objective evaluation of, and the establishment of a clear relationship with, the workload' (Executive Summary, para 22). In their study of three community trusts the VFMU attempted to establish appropriate grade profiles to match observed activity within the district nursing services involved. Equating skill mix with the performance of particular tasks by particular grades is not an uncommon approach to reviewing nursing establishments; however, the two concepts of skill mix and grade mix are essentially different (Cowley 1993, RCN 1992). Staff profiles and patient outcomes are likely to differ depending on whether skill mix or grade mix is implemented.

Skill mix versus grade mix

Gibbs *et al.* (1991) have also suggested that there is a clear distinction to be made between skill mix and grade mix. Grade mix is held to be concerned with grades of staff, their costs and activities, while skill mix involves an assessment of needs, skills and outcomes. Grade mix in line with the notion of factory production assumes that there are clear boundaries attached to the work carried out by particular workers. As with the production line, an assumption is made that the job does not vary, that it is predictable and particular skills associated with particular grades once identified will be sufficient in all circumstances. The task analysis approach adopted by the

VFMU reflected this way of thinking (NHSME 1992). A range of nursing tasks was identified and suggestions were made as to which grade of staff would best be suited to perform them. The researchers suggested that eye drops could be administered by a nursing auxiliary, assuming this to be a simple procedure. What is not discussed is whether on a particular day an auxiliary would be able to recognise and respond urgently to a sudden manifestation of acute glaucoma where delay in accessing treatment could result in permanent loss of sight for the patient. Kitson (1991) cites level of knowledge as a distinguishing feature between professional and lay carers.

The task analysis approach and activity sampling assumes that nursing is a simple practice, and negates professional judgements (Cowley 1993). It makes assumptions about the nature of assessment, earmarking it as a discrete one-off activity rather than as an ongoing process that accompanies every nursing action albeit silently. Coomber *et al.* (1992) attempted to demonstrate this silent work by asking different grades of community nurses to make diary entries about their visits. It was apparent that the Commcare system used to record nursing activity in the district concerned failed to reflect the range of activity identified by the nurses themselves (from the highest to lowest grades), one of the most significant omissions being the failure to capture the high levels of assessment taking place, particularly by the G grades.

Expert practitioners

The range of simultaneous activity recorded by the higher grades in Coomber *et al.*'s study accords with Benner's (1984) notion that expert nurses are able to assimilate whole situations in a glance, to see beyond what is immediately obvious and to respond rapidly to complex and multi-faceted needs (Cowley 1993). This ability is in contrast with the novice who relies on rule-based behaviour, working in a logical, linear mode and dealing only with the immediate presenting situation. Paradoxically this limited way of working appears to be more easily captured during task analysis which adopts a cross-sectional rather than a longitudinal approach. The snap-shot methodology captures the present but not the future. For example, conversation not directly related to a task in hand might be described as having no nursing purpose when recorded objectively by an outside observer.

The Value for Money Unit (VFMU) (NHSME 1992) divided the activity of talking to patients into general/social and condition-related. Cowley (1993) has illustrated the artificiality of this division in her example from practice. Cowley described how when visiting with a DN specialist practice teacher, the latter related a conversation with a patient in the early stages of a terminal illness whose physical needs for care were not yet great. The specialist teacher, in an attempt to establish an opening into the subject of dying, commented on a religious text on the wall. The short remark resulted in an exchange about God and belief, not immediately relevant to the visit in hand but of enormous significance for care to be delivered at a later date. It would be interesting to know how the agency nurses recruited to collect data for the VFMU study (NHSME 1992) would have recorded the conversation that was not directly related to the patient's present condition. The quality of care delivered in the last stages of life can depend very much on earlier seemingly irrelevant conversations.

The snap-shot approach is problematic because it does not reveal what is being missed or what is of value for the future. A less skilled nurse may have managed adequately in that visit to all intents and purposes to the outside observer. The practitioner in Cowley's example was able to anticipate the patient's long-term needs, yet this skilled intervention was made to look simple and effortless. Nonetheless the VFMU felt able on the basis of their study to recommend changes in the community nursing profile, valuing the management function of G and H grade community nurses and seeing the need for these nurses to concentrate their activities on assessment.

Separation of assessment from the delivery of care, as advocated by the VFMU, causes difficulty for the nursing profession. Caring is held to be fundamental to promoting, creating and restoring health (Cowley 1993). Caring has been described as a dynamic therapeutic function that depends on the context (Dunlop 1986). It is has been described as intensely intimate, emotional and personal and cannot be delegated (Cowley 1993). In the eyes of some, attempts to reduce it to a set of behaviours that can be observed, counted or measured deserve criticism (Northcott & Bayntun Lees 1993). Caring may involve technical and practical assistance but it also has psychological and social aspects that include empathy, understanding, warmth, mutual trust and belief, insight into the meaning of the situation and giving time (Cowley 1993). Implementation of skill and grade mix, however, demands that the caring function is to all intents and purposes delegated, thus in the eyes of many undermining the therapeutic potential of interactions. Such views rely on the judgement that unqualified staff are unable to interact with patients on a therapeutic level.

Therapeutic care and qualified staff

Evidence for the argument that registered nurses by dint of their training and education are the only nursing staff that can deliver therapeutic care is equivocal. The nature of many of the cases that are presented before the UKCC professional conduct committee would contradict any reified view of the trained nurse (UKCC 1992). Coomber *et al.* (1992) demonstrated that higher grades of community staff engaged in a larger number of activities at each visit, but, interestingly the researchers also recorded that it was the unqualified staff who recognised carers' needs most obviously. Koch and Webb (1996) on the other hand found care to be routinised and task oriented when carried out by unqualified staff. As these authors report, the literature continually questions the use of untrained personnel but Koch and Webb also point to the effects of ward culture on the care delivered. In her doctoral thesis, Thomas (1992) also highlighted the importance of culture in the delivery of care by both qualified and unqualified nurses.

Thomas (1992) compared the contribution to patient care of nursing auxiliaries with that of registered nurses using a qualitative indicator, nurse–patient interaction. Different grades of nursing staff were also compared in terms of activities performed and perceptions of their work environment. The study showed that nursing auxiliaries are capable of providing therapeutic care for elderly patients within a pattern of ward organisation which facilitates sustained nursing staff allocation and appropriate supervision and direction by registered nurses working with nursing auxiliaries. Thomas found a greater amount of therapeutic communication regardless of staff grade in wards where primary care nursing was the organisational mode. Carr-Hill *et al.* (1992) also found support for the benefits of primary nursing but questioned whether elements contained within particular organisational modes also affected care delivery. In earlier research Kitson (1991) found that the therapeutic approach of the ward sister was an indirect predictor of the quality of care in the ward. Other researchers though (Norman *et al.* 1994), were unable to support Kitson's findings (1991) possibly because changes in the organisation of nursing work had superseded many of the issues addressed by Kitson's original data collection instrument. One of these organisational changes has been the spread of primary nursing.

Primary nursing and the nursing auxiliary

Primary nursing has been defined as:

> 'a mode of nursing organisation at the unit level in which one registered nurse is designated as the primary nurse for a small number of patients upon their admission and for the duration of their stay in that unit; the primary nurse takes responsibility for planning and evaluating all aspects of their nursing care.'

> (Giovannetti 1981 cited by Thomas 1993, p. 45)

From the literature Thomas (1993) described two opposing viewpoints on the role and function of the nursing auxiliary in primary nursing. According to the first, auxiliaries should not be involved in direct patient care but support qualified staff in preparing equipment and performing domestic non-nursing duties (Pearson 1988, Macguire 1989, MacMahon 1989). Others, such as Pembrey (1985), concede that there is a role for the auxiliary in direct care for the patient whose condition is stable, under the direction of the qualified nurse.

Spitzer (1976, cited in Hockey 1978) has described the professional as a decision-maker and the auxiliary as an implementer. In this analysis, patient condition in terms of stability and the frequency of need for reassessment, would determine input from different grades of staff. Thomas (1992) suggested a ratio of one qualified staff member to one auxiliary for the elderly wards in which her study took place. Hockey (1978) described the need for clinical areas to work out the level of staffing required by delineating a danger zone which would signal the point at which the level of responsibility for decision-making was passing from qualified to unqualified staff.

Successful deployment of skill mix would therefore need as a prerequisite a detailed assessment of patient need matched with the assessment of staff skills as opposed to staff grades. Some researchers, notably Carr-Hill *et al.* (1992), have argued that levels of training mean that it is possible to equate grade with specific skills. This argument would hold water if employers were consistent in their staff profiles but different grades are afforded to people with similar levels of expertise, varying with the employing trust. In addition the ethos of professional development, as outlined in the UKCC's requirements for post registration education and practice (UKCC 1994), centres around the individual's responsibility for skills acquisition. Inevitably individuals will develop at different rates and the disparity between grade and skill is likely to become even greater.

Delegation

Detailed assessments of both patient need and staff skills thus appear to be pre-requisites to successful delegation. Of equal importance though is the wide ranging knowledge of common conditions that allows detailed instructions to be given to less experienced staff of what and when to report back. The problem of the auxiliary who fails to recognise an urgent need for treatment for glaucoma is alleviated if the potential for the condition is recognised at assessment and the trained nurse provides in the care plan careful instructions regarding signs and symptoms of concern. The problem is to decide to what degree practice is predictable. To claim that it is always so unpredictable as to require only highly qualified personnel seems as unrealistic as to suggest that it is so predictable that trained nurses are no longer required. If practice is always so unpredictable and complex some might argue that only medical consultants and not nurses should see patients, never mind unqualified staff. Perhaps eyedrops should only be administered by a senior ophthalmologist. The level of decision-making required at assessment suggests that expert registered nurses will have their place in future systems of health care delivery.

Linked to assessment and report back instructions is the need for training of unqualified staff. Without direct input into training schemes, such as those advocated by the Care Consortium and providing National Vocational Qualifications (NVQs), nurses are unlikely to feel comfortable delegating and remaining accountable for care delivered. Some who have been involved in training of unqualified staff have expressed the view that it approximates to teaching their own assassins (Keys 1997). To deny that health care assistants will increasingly usurp the traditional tasks of nursing would be naive given the historical development of nursing. The nineteenth century physician would undoubtedly be amazed to learn that district nurses in 1997 are considered by some of their general practitioner colleagues to be more knowledgeable in wound care products than themselves (Luker *et al.* 1997). What needs to be debated is whether patients, doctors or nurses have suffered as a result of the division of labour called nursing, or whether a more flexible response to health care ensued. In a study of skill mix issues in health visiting (Keys 1997), many of those who had gone down the road of embracing new ways of working reported greater effectiveness and ability to respond to client need.

If there is a belief that expert nursing is largely intuitive and that the knowledge is acquired predominantly through doing (Benner 1984), many health care assistants will also acquire levels of expertise that approximate to that of the trained nurse, just as nurses did when physicians started to relinquish tasks to them.

Attempts over the years by some in the medical profession to restrict the growth of nursing have clearly proved to have been unsuccessful. Garmanikow (1991) has chronicled some of the extreme disquiet among the medical profession about the division of labour between medicine and nursing at the end of the last century and the beginning of this one. As Garmanikow (1991) relates, the division was fraught with tension precisely because it was impossible to state at which point doctoring ended and nursing began. At the end of the day advances in medicine and the increasing complexities of modern life ensured that there was plenty for all to do.

Workman (1996), in her study of health care assistants, noted a similar tension around boundaries of work between nurses and unqualified staff. There appears to have been uncertainty on both sides but a more satisfied and committed worker resulted when there was close supervision and specifically delegated tasks. Workman (1996) also found that the relationship between qualified and unqualified staff appeared to influence the amount and type of support the unqualified worker could offer. Recommendations from the study included an increase in registered nurses' knowledge and awareness of their accountability in delegation and supervision of support workers, as well as an understanding of the principles of NVQ assessment and NVQ criteria. It is apparent from this study that the utility of the unqualified health care assistant is closely linked to characteristics and attitudes of qualified staff and the extent to which nurses are prepared to assume a supervisory role.

Conclusion

From Sarah Gamp to health care assistant history goes full circle in carving out the supervisory role of the trained nurse. Advances in medical care, combined with the need to supervise the handywomen and servants who had traditionally cared for the sick, created the need for the professional nurse in the nineteenth century. Similar forces prevail today. Pressures from medicine in terms of reducing junior doctor hours (DoH 1991) impinge on nursing, as it is perceived that in the time-honoured tradition nurses can expand their roles and assume those tasks that doctors discard. At the same time an ageing population with high levels of chronic illness is likely also to demand attention from the nursing profession. These pressures are present against a backdrop of cost containment in health care.

Ideally nurses would like to feel that all those who need nursing care would receive it from registered nurses who combine knowledge and humanity to achieve the best therapeutic outcomes for patients. Yet in seemingly less pressured times it has been unqualified staff who have delivered the greater part of hands-on care, particularly in the case of the elderly. In itself this might be considered argument enough for an all trained workforce, given the past poor reputation of elderly care nursing.

Nonetheless, the historical shortfall in recruitment to nursing shows little sign of being reversed so even if there were the economic resources to consider an all trained workforce, the candidates are unlikely to present themselves in sufficient numbers. Dingwall *et al.* (1988) have also pointed out that the aspirations of the profession have rarely prevailed against political, economic and social exigency.

Further, the lack of interest displayed by the profession in the development of the support worker means that their potential to deliver high quality care cannot yet be validly assessed. Encouragingly the evidence suggests that the qualified nurse is pivotal in creating the environment in which all grades of staff, trained and untrained, are able to deliver therapeutic care. Rigid adherence to a belief in a hands-on role alone at the expense of this more managerial function will deny patients access to good quality of care, as demographic trends and policy suggest that some people will have to continue to receive care from unqualified personnel. In looking forward to the magical day when all patients will be nursed by qualified staff, the profession has been prepared to allow many to receive care from those who have worked without appropriate delegation, supervision and training because all would be all right in the end when only professional nurses occupied the field.

The dangers, however, in embracing the support worker are all too evident. There are those who advocate drastic reductions in the nursing workforce (Caines 1993). Consequently situations could arise where appropriate delegation is no longer possible, with untrained staff entering that danger zone outlined earlier (Hockey 1978) where decision-making falls to those without the requisite knowledge. Nonetheless the profession should take heart in looking to its origins. History suggests that the need for the qualified nurse as supervisor would become as apparent as it did in the last century. Unqualified workers have survived despite attempts by the profession to exclude them from nursing. They will not go away now. Support workers have much to offer both to patients and to registered nurses. The latter, however, need to understand their own managerial functions in terms of accountability, teaching and delegation and must be prepared to share a therapeutic philosophy.

References

Abel-Smith, B. (1960) *A History of the Nursing Profession.* Heinneman, London.

Adams, G.F. & McIllwraith, P.L. (1963) *Geriatric Nursing: A Study of the Work of Geriatric Ward Staff.* Oxford University Press, London.

Ahmed, L. & Kitson, A. (1993) Complementary roles of nurse and health care assistant. *Journal of Clinical Nursing,* 2, 287–97.

Alexander, Z. & Dewjee, A. (eds) (1984) *Wonderful Adventures of Mrs Seacole in Many Lands.* Falling Wall Press, Bristol.

Audit Commission (1991) *The virtue of patients: making best use of ward nursing resources.* National Health Service Report No 4. HMSO, London.

Audit Commission (1992) *Homeward Bound: a new course for community nursing.* HMSO, London.

Benner, P. (1984) *From Novice to Expert, Excellence and Power in Clinical Nursing Practice.* Addison Wesley, Menlo Park, CA.

Boulton, A. (1996) Nursing shortfall hits Britain. *British Medical Journal,* 312, 139.

Bowling, A., Farquhar, M. & Grundy, E. (1993) Who are the consistently high users of health and social services? A follow-up study two and a half years later of people aged 85+ at baseline. *Health & Social Care,* 1, 277–87.

Buchan, J. (1997) Heading for a double whammy. *Nursing Standard,* **11**(21), 24–5.

Caines, E. (1993) Amputation is crucial to the nation's health. *The Guardian,* 11 May.

Carr-Hill, R., Dixon, P., Gibbs, I., Griffiths, M., Higgins, M., McCaughan & Wright, K.M. (1992) *Skill Mix and the Effectiveness of Nursing Care.* Centre for Health Economics, University of York, York.

Central Statistical Office (1996) *Social Trends.* HMSO, London.

Coomber, R., Cubbin, J., Davison, N. & Pearson, P. (1992) *Nursing Skillmix Review.* Newcastle Community Health.

Cowley, S. (1993) Skill mix: value for whom? *Health Visitor,* **66**(5), 166–71.

Davies, S.M. (1992) Consequences of the division of nursing labour for elderly patients in a continuing care setting. *Journal of Advanced Nursing,* 17, 582–9.

Day, M. (1994) Degree-level entry 'is vital' to boost nursing image. *Nursing Times,* **90**(43), 26 October, 11.

Department of Health (1991) *The Calman Report: Junior Doctors – the New Deal.* NHSME, London.

DHSS (1972) *Report of the Committee on Nursing* (Chairman Asa Briggs). Cmnd 5115. HMSO, London.

DHSS (1987) *The Role and Preparation of Support Workers to Nurses, Midwives and Health Visitors and the Implications for Manpower and Service Planning.* DHSS, London.

Dickson, N. & Cole, A. (1987) Nurse's little helper? *Nursing Times,* **83**(10), 24–6.

Dingwall, R., Rafferty, A.M. & Webster, C. (1988) *An Introduction to the Social History of Nursing.* Routledge, London.

Dunlop, M. (1986) Is a science of caring possible? *Journal of Advanced Nursing,* 11, 611–70.

Fries, J.F. (1980) Ageing, natural death and the compression of morbidity. *New England Journal of Medicine,* 303, 130–35.

Fries, J.F. (1996) Physical activity, the compression of morbidity, and the health of the elderly. *Journal of the Royal Society of Medicine,* 89, 64–8.

Garmanikow, E. (1991) Nurse or woman: gender and professionalism in reformed nursing 1860–1923. In: *Anthropology and Nursing* (eds P. Holden & J. Littlewood). Routledge, London.

Gibbs, I., McCaughan, D. & Griffiths, M. (1991) Skill mix in nursing: a selected review of the literature. *Journal of Advanced Nursing*, 16, 242–9.

Giovanetti, P. (1981) A comparative study of team and primary nursing care. Unpublished PhD thesis, Johns Hopkins University. Baltimore, Ma. In: Comparing Qualified Nurse and Auxiliary Roles (1993, L. Thomas). *Nursing Times*, **89**(38), 22 September, 45–8.

Gruenberg, E.M. (1977) The failures of success. Millbank Memorial Fund Q55 3-24, cited in The Epidemiology of Ageing (1992, E. Grundy). In: *Textbook of Gerontology and Geriatric Medicine*, (eds J. Brocklehurst, R. Tallis & H. Fillit), (4th edn), pp. 1–20. Churchill Livingstone, Edinburgh.

Hardie, M. (1978) Auxiliaries: who needs them? A case study in nursing. In: *Nursing Auxiliaries In Health Care*, (eds M. Hardie & L. Hockey). Croom Helm, London.

Hawthorne, M.H. & Hickson, M.E. (1993) Improving outcomes in patients with heart failure. In: *Key Aspects of Caring for the Acutely Ill*, (eds S.G. Funk, E.M. Tornquist, M.T. Champagne & R.A. Wiese). Springer, New York.

Health Services Management Unit (1996) *The Future Healthcare Workforce*. The Steering Group Report, Health Services Management Unit, University of Manchester.

Henderson, V. (1966) *The Nature of Nursing*. Macmillan, New York.

Heslop, A.P. & Bagnall, P. (1988) A study to evaluate the intervention of a nurse visiting patients with disabling chest disease in the community. *Journal of Advanced Nursing*, 13, 71–7.

Hockey, L. (1978) Nursing auxiliaries – the economic argument. In: *Nursing Auxiliaries in Health Care*, (eds M. Hardie & L. Hockey). Croom Helm, London.

Hunt, G. & Wainwright, P. (eds) (1994) *Expanding the Role of the Nurse: The Scope of Professional Practice*. Blackwell Science, Oxford.

ICN (1993) *Nursing Support Workers Position Statement and Guidelines*. International Council of Nurses, Geneva.

Keys, M. (1997) Health visitors' reactions to implementing skill mix. *Nursing Standard*, **11**(21), 34–5.

Kitson, A.L. (1991) *Therapeutic Nursing and the Hospitalised Elderly*. Scutari Press, London.

Koch, T. & Webb, C. (1996) The biomedical construction of ageing: implications for nursing care of older people. *Journal of Advanced Nursing*, 23, 954–9.

Leifer, D. (1996) Recruitment crisis. *Nursing Standard*, **10**(15), 18–19.

Lister, P. (1997) The art of nursing in a 'postmodern' context. *Journal of Advanced Nursing*, 25, 38–44.

Luker, K., Austin, L., Hogg, C., Ferguson, B. & Smith, K. (1997) Over-the-counter items bought by a sample of community nurse patients. *British Journal of Community Health Nursing*, **2**(2), 69–74.

Macguire, J. (1989) Prime movers. *Nursing the Elderly*, September, 9, 19–24.

MacMahon, R. (1989) One to one. *Nursing Times*, **85**(2), 39–40.

Majeed, A. (1993) *Ischaemic heart disease in Wandsworth–implications for purchasers.* Unpublished report for the Department of Public Health Medicine, Wandsworth Health Authority.

Manton, K.G. (1982) Changing concepts of morbidity and mortality in the elderly population. Millbank Memorial Fund Q55, cited in The Epidemiology of Ageing (1992, E. Grundy). In: *Textbook of Gerontology and Geriatric Medicine* (eds J. Brocklehurst, R. Tallis & H. Fillit), (4th Edition) pp. 1–20. Churchill Livingstone, Edinburgh.

Masiello Millar, M. (1994) Current trends in the primary care management of chronic congestive heart failure. *Nurse Practitioner*, **19**(5), 64–70.

McKenna, H. (1995) Nursing skill mix substitutions and quality of care: an exploration of assumptions from the research literature. *Journal of Advanced Nursing*, 21, 452–9.

McKeown, M. (1995) The transformation of nurses' work. *Journal of Nursing Management*, 3, 67–73.

Mersey Regional Health Authority (1989) *Job Satisfaction*. Mersey RHA, Liverpool.

MoH (Ministry of Health) Board of Education (1939) *Inter-Departmental Committee on Nursing Services Interim Report* (Chairman: The Earl of Athlone). HMSO, London.

Moody, H.R. (1995) Ageing, Meaning and the Allocation of Resources. *Ageing and Society*, 15, 163–84.

Murphy, R. (1988) *Social Closure: The Theory of Monopolisation and Exclusion*. Clarendon Press, London.

NHSME (National Health Service Management Executive) Value for Money Unit (1992) *Skillmix in the District Nursing Service*. HMSO, London.

Nolan, P. (1993) *A History of Mental Health Nursing*. Chapman Hall, London.

Nolan, M.R. & Grant, G. (1989) Addressing the needs of informal carers: a neglected area of nursing practice. *Journal of Advanced Nursing*, 14, 950–61.

Norman, I.J., Redfern, S.J., Tomalin, D.A. & Oliver, S. (1994) Kitson's therapeutic nursing function indicator as a predictor of the quality of nursing care in hospital wards. *International Journal of Nursing Studies*, **31**(2), 109-18.

Northcott, N. & Bayntun-Lees, D. (1993) Who cares? *Nursing Times*, **89**(22), 40–41.

Pearson, A. (1988) *Primary Nursing*. Croom Helm, Beckenham.

Pearson, M. & Wistow, G. (1995) The boundary between health care and social care. *British Medical Journal*, 311, 208–209.

Pembrey, S. (1985) A framework for care. *Nursing Times*, **81**(50), 47–9.

Phillips, S. (1988) *Consequences of the division of nursing labour for elderly patients in a continuing care setting*. Unpublished MSc thesis, University of Surrey, Guildford.

Ramprogus, V. (1995) *The Deconstruction of Nursing*. Avebury, Aldershot.

Roberts, J. (1996) British Nurses at War 1914–1918: ancillary personnel and the battle for registration. *Nursing Research*, **45**(3), 167–9.

Robinson, J., Stillwell, J., Hawley, C. & Hempstead, N. (1989) *The Role of the Support Worker in the Ward Health Care Team*. Nursing Policy Studies 6. Nursing Policy Studies Centre and Health Services Research Unit, University of Warwick.

Rogers, C.R. (1969) *Freedom to Learn*. Merrill, Ohio.

Royal College of Nursing (RCN) (1992) *Skill Mix and Reprofiling: a Guide for Members*. RCN, London.

Rye, D. (1978) Nursing auxiliaries: a professional perspective in relation to role and subsequent training. In: *Nursing Auxiliaries in Health Care*, (eds M. Hardie & L. Hockey). Croom Helm, London.

Salvage, J. (1988) In the ghetto. *Nursing Times*, **84**(32), 22.

Seccombe, I. (1996) Just a little local difficulty? *Nursing Standard*, **10**(19), 24–5.

Seymour, J. (1992) Pick and mix. *Nursing Times*, **88**(33), 12 August, 19.

Skeet, M. (1978) Division of labour: roles, responsibilities and accountability within the team concept. In: *Nursing Auxiliaries In Health Care*, (eds M. Hardie & L. Hockey). Croom Helm, London.

Skeet, M. & Crout, E. (1977) *Health Needs Help*. Blackwell Science, Oxford.

Spitzer, W.O. (1976) The Effect of the Allied Health Professions on Cost Containing Shifts in the Provision of Health Services cited by Hockey, L. (1978) Nursing

Auxiliaries – The Economic Argument In: Hardie, M., Hockey, L. (eds) (1978) *Nursing Auxiliaries In Health Care*. Croom Helm, London.

Thomas, L. (1993) Comparing qualified nurse and auxiliary roles. *Nursing Times*, **89**(38), 45–8.

Thomas, L. (1992) *A comparison of the work of qualified nurses and nursing auxiliaries in primary, team and functioning nursing wards*. Unpublished PhD thesis, University of Newcastle upon Tyne, Newcastle upon Tyne.

Townsend, C. (1989) Employment-led qualifications for NHS support staff. *Personnel Management*, **21**(10), 60–65.

UKCC (1986) *Project 2000: A New Preparation for Practice*. UKCC, London.

UKCC (1992) Professional Conduct. *Occasional report on selected cases 1 April 1991–31 March 1992*. UKCC, London.

UKCC (1994) *The Future of Professional Practice – the Council's Standards for Education and Practice following Registration*. UKCC, London.

Waite, R. (1989) School-leaver decline and the mature labour market: options and implications. In: *Health Care UK*, (eds A. Harrison & J. Grethen). King's Fund Institute, London.

Wandelt, M. & Ager, J. (1974) *Quality Patient Care Scale*. Appleton-Century-Crofts, New York.

Wells, T. (1980) *Problems in Geriatric Nursing Care*. Churchill Livingstone, Edinburgh.

While, A.E. & Barriball, K.L. (1994) *A Study to Explore the Perceptions and Needs of Continuing Professional Education among Nurses in Practice in Two District Health Authorities in South West Thames Regional Health Authority*. Commissioned by South West Thames Regional Health Authority, King's College, London.

Workman, B.A. (1996) An investigation into how the health care assistants perceive their role as 'support workers' to qualified staff. *Journal of Advanced Nursing*, 23, 612–19.

6 The Organisation of Nursing Work

Joanne Fitzpatrick and Sally Redfern

This chapter examines different approaches to the organisation of nursing work. We describe the key characteristics of different nursing practice organisational systems and explore how much individualised patient care is a focus in each. The impact of different organisational systems is examined from the perspective of nurses, nursing practice and service users. Organisational and financial implications are noted. We draw attention to potential tensions between nursing and managerial values and urge that common ground is reached so that greater accountability, responsibility, autonomy and influence for nurses, and enhanced continuity and comprehensiveness of care, are achieved. When this happens everyone will benefit – nurses, service users and the health service.

Key characteristics of different systems of work organisation

Functional, team and primary nursing, together with multidisciplinary approaches to work organisation, are described below. Findings from a project carried out by the Nursing Research Unit, King's College, London, are used to examine the extent to which individualised patient care is a focus in each approach (Redfern 1996) and differences between the different systems are identified.

Functional nursing

Task allocation or functional nursing as a system of nursing work organisation has three characteristics: it takes a mechanistic approach with nursing work categorised into tasks (Berry & Metcalf 1986); tasks are allocated to nurses according to the perceived level of skill required to perform them (Chavasse 1981, Kron 1981, Pembrey 1975); and tasks are allocated by the nurse in charge (Durbin 1981). Thus the most senior nurse is a manager (Bowman *et al*, 1991), retaining responsibility, authority and ultimate accountability for the planning and co-ordination of care. Other nurses are delegated responsibility for performing tasks under supervision. Functional nursing is equivalent to Adams' (1996) 'centralised' nursing system, which was evident in just over a tenth (14%, 10) of the participating wards in her study, where most authority and responsibility for care was retained by ward leaders.

Team nursing

Similar to the functional nursing system, team nursing operates within a hierarchical management structure. Team nursing is popular in different practice settings (Thomas & Bond 1990; Maben *et al.* 1993). In a study of the organisation of nursing care in 27 acute and rehabilitation wards for care of the older adult, Thomas and Bond found that most ward sisters (71%) used some form of team nursing. Team nursing most closely resembles the 'two-tier' system of nursing work organisation empirically derived by Adams (1996). Under the two-tier system, the nursing team is given considerable responsibility with most vested in the team leader, but ultimate authority and accountability is retained by the ward manager. The majority of wards (76%, 56) in Adams' study had implemented a two-tier system. In team nursing, therefore, nurses are grouped and allocated to a number of patients for a period (Berry & Metcalf 1986), and the team is headed by a registered nurse who has authority for the management of patient care and responsibility for co-ordinating client care in the team (Marks-Maran 1978).

Functional and team nursing often exist alongside each other, as happens when task allocation operates within a team approach. The result can be a loss in both continuity of carer and individualised patient care (Redfern 1996). What so often happens, for all sorts of reasons, is that what is done in practice is not what is espoused. That is to say, nurses advocate a team nursing approach but find themselves resorting to functional nursing when their resources (staffing, skill-mix, etc.) are overstretched.

Investigating systems of work organisation in nursing is not easy; values underpinning a chosen organisational framework and its features are often not clearly articulated. Thomas and Bond (1990) developed a feasible method for classifying different systems of nursing work organisation which could, with benefit, be exploited in future research. Their questionnaire focuses on six discriminators:

(1)   Grouping of nurses and length of allocation to specific patients
(2)   Allocation of nursing work
(3)   Organisation of the duty rota
(4)   Nursing accountability for patient care
(5)   Responsibility for documentation of nursing care for allocated patients
(6)   Liaison with medical/paramedical staff.

Primary nursing

Primary nursing espouses a patient-centred approach to the organisation of nursing work. Its chief distinguishing feature is that individual patients are allocated a named nurse who is responsible and accountable for their care for as long as it is required. Primary nursing employs a flattened organisational structure (Adams 1996) and has built on the nursing process philosophy and work method to emphasise person-centred care (Salvage

1990, Smith 1991). It takes an individualised and holistic approach by involving patients/clients, family members and significant others (McFarlane 1976, Hunt & Marks-Maran 1986, UKCC 1992a). Mead and McGuire (1993) used a Delphi survey to identify 16 key features of primary nursing. The top four features are:

(1) Accountability, authority and responsibility for a case-load of patients
(2) Individualised patient care
(3) Case-load attachment from admission to discharge
(4) Continuity of care

Similar to Adams' (1996) 'devolved' organisational system, primary nursing enjoys a greater degree of devolved power than occurs in team and functional nursing, although ultimate authority for a client group is often retained centrally. In the late 1980s, Bowers (1989, p. 18) asserted that: 'It is even possible that it [primary nursing] may become the accepted method of nursing care organisation'. It is certainly favoured in government circles (Audit Commission 1991). However, in the 1990s a devolved primary nursing system was not common; it was operating in only 3% (19) of the wards in Mead and McGuire's (1993) study and 11% (74 wards) in Adams' study (1996). These findings underline our earlier point that what is espoused is often not practised, and nurses freely admit that they resort to team nursing as second-best because primary nursing is unrealistic (Redfern 1996).

Primary nursing is the preferred method of organising nursing work in many nursing development units. In a study of 28 Department of Health-funded nursing development units, half endorsed primary nursing or a related version such as key-working. No clinical leader advocated functional nursing, and none used team nursing, they said, except in conjunction with primary nursing. Sometimes they resorted to functional nursing when staffing was very low and workload very high (Redfern & Stevens 1998). Four (out of 17) aims of working at nursing development units identified by clinical leaders refer broadly to two of the features of primary nursing identified by Mead and McGuire (1993) mentioned earlier: accountability, authority and responsibility for a case-load of patients; and individualised patient care. The four aims are:

(1) Promote needs-led, individualised, partnership-based practice
(2) Promote excellence in practice
(3) Develop nurses' therapeutic skills
(4) Be accountable and responsible for decisions made (Redfern & Stevens 1998).

Continuity of care and case-load attachment from admission to discharge – the other two of Mead and McGuire's features – were endorsed by these nursing development units in that individual nurses were responsible for the care of several patients/clients throughout the client's stay. Many staff in these units said they were so used to primary nursing now that it had become 'automatic'.

The concept of the nursing development unit seems to be evolving into the broader 'practice development unit' (Mullen 1995) in which multi-professional team-working is the goal, given that one profession cannot meet all the needs of patients. There are also nurse-led units, some of which are hospital-based (Davies 1994, Riley 1995, Mullen 1995, Harris *et al.* 1996, Batehup *et al.* 1997) and others are based in the community; many nursing homes would fit this description, for example Nazarko (1998). Nurse-led units vary from those in which the nurse is the main co-ordinator of care and treatment to those in which nurses also take patient referrals, provide the main therapeutic activity and take responsibility for discharge decisions. The forms of nursing work organisation within these different types of units differ but many are committed to primary nursing or a close relation like key-working.

Multi-disciplinary approaches to care organisation

Examples of recent developments in patterns of multidisciplinary working are case management and patient-focused care systems. These approaches reflect 'the increased influence of the general management agenda on care provision, emphasising the need to achieve efficiency, effectiveness and enhanced productivity' (Adams 1996, p. 6) and are appealing in an economically compromised health service.

Case management has been adopted by community (Bergen 1992) and mental health services (Gournay 1995) and more recently within the acute institutional setting (Riches *et al.* 1994). The focus of this approach to work organisation is managing the path of a particular patient/client (a case, such as a patient with asthma, fractured neck of femur, suicidal behaviour) through a programme of 'managed care' (Petryshen & Petryshen, 1992). Managed care refers to systems established by either the provider or purchaser of health care who aims to ensure availability of services and resources appropriate to identified needs. There is a strong emphasis on effectiveness and efficiency (Hale 1995). Lumsdon and Hagland's (1993) discussion of a US survey of 581 health care executives (conducted by Hospitals and Health Networks and Medicus Systems Corporation, 1993) identified improvements in quality, cost savings, better teamwork and patient satisfaction as key advantages of critical paths. We examine such issues later in the chapter.

Like other systems of work organisation, case management has been interpreted and practised in different ways (Lyon 1993; Hale 1995; Waterman *et al.* 1996). Bergen (1992) found that various titles were used to describe case management in the community, including 'key-working', 'care programme approach', and 'care management'. Within acute care, Hale (1995) has identified five key features of case management:

(1) An identified case manager
(2) Multidisciplinary care maps
(3) Analysis of any deviation from the critical path

(4) Nursing documentation regarding the care process
(5) Multi-disciplinary case consultations.

Client care is co-ordinated by the case manager for as long as it is required (LeClair 1991). Care maps provide a framework for the care process and management of resources (Hale 1995). Unlike the primary nurse or team leader roles, the nurse acting as case manager does not necessarily take a clinical role (Hale 1995). All those involved in care provision accept accountability (Petryshen & Petryshen 1992) but ultimate accountability is vested in the case manager. The role of the nurse as case manager presents the opportunity for increased autonomy (Petryshen & Petryshen 1992). In Bergen's (1992) study, nurses as case managers within the community identified increased accountability and flexibility of practice as benefits of this system of work organisation.

Patient-focused care shares features of case management: cost-related; grouping of patients/clients with similar service needs; planning and delivery of care by a multidisciplinary team; and use of multidisciplinary care maps which are time-structured (Buchan 1995, Burchell & Jenner 1996). According to Burchell and Jenner (1996, p. 68), patient-focused care 'involves the decentralisation of diagnostic, therapeutic and other support services to ward units and the creation of a multi-skilled workforce of co-ordinated care teams'. Under the patient-focused care system the traditional ward sister role has been replaced by the clinical manager, although it is the care leader who co-ordinates and manages care on a day-to-day basis and is assisted by associates or care givers (usually auxiliaries) (Morgan 1993). Evaluation of the patient-focused care system of work organisation to date is limited (Buchan 1995, Humphreys 1996).

The impact of different systems of work organisation on nursing practice

Having summarised the key distinguishing features of different systems of nursing work organisation, we turn here to examine how much the different systems influence nursing practice and its quality. We consider patient-centredness, the therapeutic nurse–client relationship, management of care activities, and management of human resources.

Patient-centredness

As we have indicated, functional nursing is underpinned by a task-centred approach which tends not to be individualised or holistic care (Bendall 1973, Berry & Metcalf 1986), and is designed to satisfy medical rather than patient need (Fretwell 1980). In an early study Bendall (1973) observed task-centred care in hospital which, she maintained, militated against caring for the patient as a 'biopsychosocial being': 'the mere urgency of "getting the work done" seemed to make nurses deaf and blind to what was going on round them' (Bendall 1973, p. 37). The influence of a patient-centred versus a task-centred nursing organisational approach on the performance of 42 baccalaureate nurses was investigated by Christman (1971) in America. Using the Slater nursing competencies rating scale (Slater 1967) she found nursing performance to be significantly superior in the patient-centred setting. Her findings suggest that a patient-centred approach enhances the quality of nurse performance. She did not, though, examine the influence of other important variables (ward philosophy, leadership style, intra- and inter-professional working, staffing levels and skill mix) which could have been as important as the nursing system in affecting performance.

Continuity of care, responsibility and accountability, and good nurse-patient relationships were identified as facilitators of health education and health promotion practice by a third (46) of all ward sisters working in six case study wards in three acute hospital settings in England (Maben *et al.* 1993). The researchers stress, however, that any endeavour to introduce these facilitators, irrespective of the system of work organisation in practice, would fail unless the ward philosophy, leadership style and ward ethos are supportive.

Brown's (1989) exploratory study of task- and patient-centredness in two medical wards in a children's hospital in England revealed that, in stark contrast to the task-centred approach, the patient-centred ward sister interacted more with patients and families, used ward facilities for the benefit of patients and families, demonstrated greater awareness of the psychosocial needs of patients and others, and functioned effectively as a team member. Findings such as these suggest that functional nursing is not compatible with the principles of individualised patient care, a conclusion supported by Redfern (1996) and Vlerick (1996). The research by Redfern's team identified five key facilitators of individualised patient care:

(1) Nurses' personal qualities (e.g. believing in individualised care, possessing knowledge and experience, interpersonal skills, and leadership qualities)
(2) Organisational issues (e.g. continuity of care for patients, support for students and untrained staff, care delivery by qualified staff, supportive management)
(3) Staffing issues (e.g. adequate staffing levels and skill mix)
(4) Commitment from other health care professionals
(5) Patient characteristics (e.g. preference for partnership in care).

Under the patient-focused care system, enhanced continuity of care owing to a restricted number of staff coming into contact with patients/clients, together with an emphasis on the patient's/client's experience, are in keeping with an individualised patient care focus. However, other elements of the patient-focused care system are not compatible with individualised patient care (Redfern & Evers 1995). It can be argued, for example, that multiskilling inhibits continuity of carer and opportunities for client involvement.

Therapeutic nurse–client relationship

A predominant focus on tasks does not foster development of a therapeutic nurse-client relationship, with its emphasis on 'listening and observing as well as talking with patients' (Redfern & Evers 1995, p. 3). Indeed, nursing staff in functional wards in Thomas' (1994) study spent the least amount of time communicating with patients in comparison with their primary and team nursing counterparts. Smith (1992) found that patients highlighted attitudes and feelings rather than technical ability when asked to describe a 'good' nurse. Characteristics of the 'good' nurse were specified as kind, helpful, considerate, understanding, and able to talk with and listen to clients. It is through the use of effective communication skills that the patient is recognised and cared for as a human being with individual needs. Unlike functional nursing, a team nursing system presents much more of an opportunity for the patient/client to identify with a group of nurses and with a named nurse, if work within the team is organised using patient allocation. This approach facilitates opportunities for client involvement, partnership and empowerment (DoH 1991, UKCC 1992a, NHSME 1993).

As we have said, team nursing was regarded as 'a good second best' after primary nursing in facilitating individualised patient care (Redfern 1996). Lending support to this, Wilson-Barnett *et al.* (1995) reported that continuity of care and accountability by a named nurse within primary or team nursing is associated with good nursing care, a team spirit and a positive learning environment. Research that has attempted to compare the effects of different nursing systems on practice has drawn few firm conclusions because of the difficulty of finding wards using an unambiguous version of task, team or primary nursing. We submit, though, that it is the characteristics of primary nursing that should be investigated, such as continuity of care and accountability, and how they operate in practice rather than the system itself. This recommendation is supported by Thomas *et al.* (1996) who found that, while there was no significant difference in patient satisfaction with care between team and primary nursing wards, a significant improvement did occur when patients knew who their nurse was. The 'named nurse' concept is enshrined in the Patient's Charter (DoH 1991), which puts empowerment of the service user high on the health care agenda.

Verbal interaction has been used as an indicator of the quality of nursing practice within different organisational settings (MacGuire *et al.* 1993, Thomas 1994). Thomas (1994) found that nurses and auxiliaries working in primary nursing wards spent significantly more time communicating with patients than nurses in functional wards. Further, nurses in primary nursing wards more often offered patients choice, explained aspects of care to patients and sought feedback from patients about care delivery. 'Basic' care, such as assisting patients/clients with their activities of living (Thomas 1993), was valued as an integral component of individualised patient care to a greater extent by nurses and auxiliaries in the primary nursing wards, in contrast to the functional and team nursing wards where basic care was delegated to nursing auxiliaries.

Management of care activities

An organisational system like functional nursing, which emphasises accomplishment of tasks, may be the best way of managing certain clinical events, such as emergencies and day surgery. For such events, performing under the direction of a key authoritative figure may be the most efficient and effective approach to care management because it maximises use of available skills and resources. Clarity of role and responsibilities is a key strength of a functional system (Vlerick 1996), together with acquisition and mastery of nursing tasks. Counter-arguments, however, are that not all nursing work can be so easily defined in task-specific terms. Also, functional nursing accentuates the physical components of ill-health and espouses 'outdated and parochial conceptions of persons, health and health care' (Reed & Ground 1997, p. 150).

In contrast, an individualistic and holistic approach to care organisation recognises the biological, psychological and social needs of patients and clients (McFarlane 1976, Hunt & Marks-Maran 1986, UKCC 1992a). In this regard, functional nursing is criticised as being reductionistic and mechanical, contributing to a fragmented care approach and unmet patient/client needs (Thomas 1992). Similar criticisms are also levelled at case management and patient-focused care systems due to grouping of patients/clients according to diagnoses (Morgan 1993). Conversely, it is argued that common patient needs are identifiable and establishing a case management system or patient-focused care system enables the development and implementation of an evidence-based, inter-professional plan of care. Case management and patient-focused care systems can therefore foster a more co-ordinated approach to the care process (Jones 1995).

Management of human resources

The feasibility of adopting functional nursing to cope with increasing nursing staff shortages within the health service has been investigated (Procter 1989, 1991). Procter (1991) observed how dependence on a student nurse workforce in three wards (care of older adults, acute medicine and gynaecology) influenced the organisation and implementation of patient care. She concluded that ward leaders felt justified in resorting to task-oriented routines because they had to depend on a transient work force; it was the student nurses who made the most significant service contribution. However, the recent demise of the registered nurse certificate programmes and the resulting loss of these students as workers in the practice setting has contributed to a shortfall in staffing levels (Elkan *et al.* 1995). An expansion of the support worker role has occurred as a result. This means that nurses now work with a greater number of support workers, are accountable for the care they give, and are responsible for increasing numbers of supernumerary students. This raises concerns regarding the availability of adequate numbers of nurses to act as role models for students and support workers.

Changing to patient-centred approaches, such as primary nursing, presents challenges for achieving continuity in the allocation of nurses to patients and ensuring supervision of support workers (Procter, 1991). Adequate skill mix and staffing levels are important factors in facilitating individualised patient care (Redfern 1996), together with a more devolved system of nursing work organisation (Mead & McGuire 1993, Adams 1996). Sufficient human resources, especially the need for adequate skill mix and staffing levels, are essential pre-requisites for individualised patient care. Devolving responsibility for acquiring nursing resources to nurses at ward level can be effective in ensuring that such requirements are secured. Salvage (1985) has argued that it is unreasonable to hold nurses accountable for their care-giving when they do not have authority within the health care system to control resource allocation. The UK situation contrasts with Tahan's (1993) US study which underlined the control of finances and resource allocation as an important role of the nurse case manager.

The need for authority is confirmed in a study of clinical leadership in nursing development units, many of which use primary nursing (Christian & Norman 1998). The success with which nurses can act as effective and influential clinical leaders depends on their position in the organisational hierarchy. Clinical leaders without line management responsibility are free to develop a visionary strategy for their unit but do not carry the authority needed to implement the strategy. Those with line management responsibility are so caught up in day-to-day administrative concerns that they have no opportunity to develop, or even think about, strategy. The most successful approach is to divide responsibility for strategic development and day-to-day management between two joint leaders. This works well as long as the two leaders have a good working relationship.

Procter (1995) cautions against using transient staff (agency and bank nurses) to minimise the disabling effects of inadequate grade mix and staffing levels. Transient staff were employed for 59% of the shifts she observed over a nine-week period. The difficulties for clinical managers of ensuring continuity of carer in nursing practice are clear from work such as Procter's. There are concerns, too, for professional socialisation of nursing students who have to be found suitable clinical placements (Jowett *et al.* 1994, White *et al.* 1994).

Other recent developments in nursing such as role extension to reduce junior doctors' working hours (Bradshaw 1995, Dowling *et al.* 1995) also influence organisation of nursing work. Such developments have been received enthusiastically by some but cautiously by others. Sceptics fear that non-specialist nurses will become de-skilled and care will be fragmented. They criticise what they see to be an erosion of the nursing role (Garbett 1996a). On the other hand, supporters see opportunities arising from these developments, such as expansion of the nursing role and advancement of the nursing profession (Shiell *et al.* 1993). This is reflected in the UKCC's *Scope of Professional Practice* document (UKCC 1992b), the essence of which is continued practice development and specialist nursing. As Mills (1996) has discussed, advanced nursing practice (e.g. roles such as consultant nurse, nurse practitioner and nurse-led clinics) is more than a collection of extended roles. Rather, the specialist practitioner 'will be the team leader, role model and facilitator of innovative and creative practice in response to patient/client need' (Wallace & Gough 1995, p. 942). Issues surrounding professional development, including the concept of advanced practice, are examined in Chapter 7.

The impact of different systems of work organisation on practitioners

Cavanagh's (1992) study with 221 female nurses in the USA found participation in decision-making at work to be positively related to job satisfaction. Since devolved decision-making is a key feature of primary nursing it is reasonable to expect nurses' satisfaction at work to be a positive outcome of primary nursing. Other research, though, has not supported this expectation, finding no difference in work satisfaction between nurses working in primary nursing and team nursing systems (Parasuraman *et al.* 1982, Wilson & Dawson 1989). Wilson and Dawson's (1989) longitudinal, quasi-experimental study also revealed no differences in sickness-absence and staff turnover between primary and team nursing cohorts. The study of nursing development units, half of which practised primary nursing, reported more sickness-absence in their staff compared to matched units that did not have nursing development unit status (Redfern *et al.* 1997). It was absences of four days or more that were largely responsible for the difference. Perhaps nursing development unit status puts an extra burden on staff – greater workload, high expectations, professional isolation, continually being in the limelight, for example – so that they succumb to illness. It would be interesting to repeat the observations to see if the rate of sickness-absence flattens out as nursing development units mature and become commonplace.

Parasuraman *et al.* (1982) found no significant difference between primary and team nursing units on perceived stress, organisational commitment, withdrawal cognition (thoughts of leaving the job) and intention to resign. Vlerick (1996) was surprised to find that nurses who worked in a system of patient assignment in a hospital in Belgium experienced emotional exhaustion and feelings of depersonalisation. He found, though, that nurses working within a functional system of organisation in another hospital also experienced emotional exhaustion and depersonalisation. Vlerick proposed five contributing factors to explain the unexpected findings from the patient-assignment group:

(1) Lack of or inability to apply psychosocial skills
(2) Lack of professional skills
(3) Inadequate social support and guidance from head nurses

(4) Insufficient support, guidance and monitoring from top management
(5) Not enough time to practise individualised care.

By contrast, other research has reported positive outcomes for nurses working under a devolved organisational system (Sellick *et al.* 1983, Reed 1988, Thomas 1992, MacGuire *et al.* 1993, Adams 1996, Webb & Pontin 1996). Nurses and students in MacGuire *et al.*'s (1993) study, for example, increased their communication with patients after primary nursing was introduced. They also enjoyed greater responsibility for patient care and job satisfaction overall. Similarly, the nurses in Webb and Pontin's (1996) study reported increased responsibility following the introduction of primary nursing, together with greater control and confidence, enhanced continuity of care, improved planning and prioritisation of care, and more effective nurse–patient relationships. Thomas (1992) found that qualified nurses in primary nursing wards perceived themselves as having significantly greater autonomy, supervisor support and physical support than their team and functional counterparts. Further, they perceived less work pressure and greater involvement and innovation than their counterparts in team nursing wards. Similarly, community nurses in Bergen's (1992) study reported increased accountability, flexibility and motivation when working under a system of case management. Control exerted by management was greater for nurses in functional nursing than in primary nursing wards in Thomas' (1992) study. It also emerged that nursing auxiliaries in the primary nursing wards perceived their work in the same way as their qualified colleagues. That is to say, perceptions of work satisfaction and pressures were similar for nurses and auxiliaries within the same mode of work organisation but there were differences between modes.

It is likely that support from managers and supervisors in encouraging nursing staff development and innovative practice, cohesion among nurses, and attention to structural factors helped to explain the greater perceived autonomy and lower work pressure of the primary nursing wards. The lack of managerial support for the Belgian nurses in Vlerick's (1996) study was probably responsible for some of this stress. Adams (1996) confirmed these factors as strengthening nurses' clinical autonomy and influence. She reported a significant association between hierarchical 'centralised nursing' and both autonomy and influence, with nurses operating the 'devolved' system achieving the highest mean score for autonomy compared to those working the 'centralised' and 'two-tier' systems. She also found autonomy and influence to be positively associated with nurses' job satisfaction. Such findings suggest that the devolved system encourages greater accountability, responsibility and autonomy for practitioners.

McMahon's (1990) study lends further support to this and identifies potential constraints associated with the system of team nursing, such as the introduction of hierarchies by imposing another level of management into a ward team (Garbett 1996b). McMahon (1990) examined power and collegial relations among nurses in four wards in two British hospitals. One ward from each hospital used primary nursing and the other two wards operated a hierarchical management structure (a single hierarchy in one and team nursing in the other). McMahon observed power to be a major component in the communication process in the team nursing ward, with nurses lower in the hierarchy regularly seeking direction and only reluctantly making independent decisions. He concluded that team nursing is just as hierarchical as the traditional management system. Further, complex communication channels were evident in the team nursing ward and intra-professional communication in both hierarchical wards was significantly less collaborative than in primary nursing wards.

Findings like these lend support to Thomas' (1992) proposition that within each system of organisation exists a culture which influences all staff. The predominant approach in all primary nursing wards in her study was to provide individualised and holistic care through continuity of nurse–patient allocation. Nurses and auxiliaries therefore adopted a multifocal (i.e. addressing the biopsychosocial domains) approach to care delivery in order to meet patients' needs comprehensively. By contrast, nurses and auxiliaries on functional and team nursing wards emphasised the distinction between 'basic' and 'technical' work, with the former being judged second-rate and therefore delegated to auxiliaries.

Implications for nurse learners' and practitioners' continuing professional development

The impact of different systems of work organisation on factors such as practitioners' job satisfaction, sickness-absence, turnover and professional issues such as responsibility and autonomy has been explored. The influence of these systems on the professional development of students and practitioners has been examined in the literature, although only to a limited extent. Only one small study was located which examined the influence of team and primary nursing on nursing students in a UK hospital (Lidbetter 1990). Two key findings were that students in the primary nursing ward relied less on the nurse-in-charge for information and support, and mentors in the primary nursing ward were more inclined to teach students. Encouraging 'life-long learning' in students is a priority for nursing's statutory bodies so that nurses can effectively manage change in health and social care provision (ENB 1994). This view is supported by Phillips *et al.* (1993) who regard continued research and education as the best means of refining and developing professional judgement. A framework to support these needs is essential, a key element of which is adequate supervision and teaching of students by nurses in the practice setting.

A functional system of work organisation, while facilitating the development and refinement of skills in nursing tasks (Vlerick 1996), is less likely to facilitate innovation, independent thinking, and the ability to influence decisions made. Thus it is limiting in its account of the ways in which the professional could develop (Reed & Ground 1997). Further, Thomas (1992) has argued that functional nursing does not advance the professional status of nursing because the area in which nurses can make a unique contribution – basic care – tends to be delegated to nursing auxiliaries. Reed and Ground (1997, p. 149) support this argument by levelling 'practical, political and philosophical' criticisms against functional nursing or 'old nursing'. A functional system does not encourage a critically reflective approach to practice which is central to effective assessment, planning, implementation and evaluation of care (Field 1987, Fish *et al.* 1991, Shamian 1991). Further, reflective activity enhances self-evaluation and the effectiveness of learning (Schön 1983, Saylor 1990) and helps nurses to identify inadequate routinised practice and instigate strategies to redress this (Dewing 1990).

Functional nursing militates against the use of reflective practice. In addition, decision-making in functional nursing is, to a large extent, vested in the nurse-in-charge through whom all communication is processed, and who adopts a gate-keeping role. The potential for inter-professional collaboration, therefore, is impaired. Inter-professional collaboration, together with clinical autonomy and influence, has been identified as necessary for individualised patient care (Adams 1996, Redfern 1996). In contrast, individual nurses operating in a system of team nursing are supported by colleagues within the team and in particular by the team leader who has responsibility for staff support and development (Garbett 1996b). Therefore a strategy to enhance professional development through a process of critical reflection is possible, although a progressive and reflective approach to practice is not a natural outcome of team nursing bearing in mind that, as we mentioned earlier, task allocation may operate within a team approach.

It is recognised that there is a need for self-monitoring and improvement of professional knowledge and clinical skills through a process of continuing professional education, augmented by awareness and application of research to practice. Uptake of continuing education is no greater in nursing development units compared to 'progressive' units without NDU status, but uptake is a good deal greater in these units compared to 'general' nursing populations (Redfern *et al.* 1997). Professional development in terms of staff appraisal and clinical supervision is also similar in nursing development units and their matched comparisons, and is significantly associated with job satisfaction (Redfern *et al.* 1997). Two-thirds of responding staff in both kinds of unit participated in appraisal meetings with a supervisor/manager, compared with only two-fifths of the staff in a study by Barriball and While (1995). Clinical supervision is more common in mental health and midwifery units than in other specialities. Regular supervision for midwives is a statutory requirement, of course. The higher level in mental health suggests that clinical supervision is becoming an established part of everyday practice, as advocated by *Working in Partnership* (Butterworth 1994).

Outcomes for service users

Positive outcomes for nurses are likely to benefit patients/clients. The study by MacGuire *et al.* (1993), conducted within an elderly care ward, reported that primary nursing was associated with positive outcomes for patients:

- An increase in the number of discharges home
- An increase in the number of clients eligible for full rehabilitation on discharge
- More patients being discharged at lower dependency rates
- More discharges under 20 days
- Less demand for support services on discharge

The death rate was also lower in comparison with the other two wards which operated team nursing. Re-admission rates remained unchanged.

A questionnaire survey of 85 patients in the study revealed no difference in perceived quality of nursing care in the primary nursing ward compared with the other wards. We note, though, that only 38% (85 out of 225) of the patients responded, so limiting the generalisability of the findings. Patient satisfaction scales which have been tested rigorously for reliability and validity were used by Thomas *et al.* (1996) to investigate the influence of primary nursing on patient satisfaction ($n = 1559$, 75% response rate). No significant differences emerged in patients' satisfaction scores or their experiences in wards operating primary nursing compared with team nursing wards. However, it was found that, irrespective of the system of nursing work organisation, patients who had identified one nurse in charge of their care reported significantly more positive experiences of nursing and were also significantly more satisfied with their nursing care, than those who could not identify their nurse. Positive outcomes for service users were also reported in Shiell *et al.*'s (1993) Australian study which evaluated the role of the case manager within a programme of care for elderly patients with fractured hip, using a before-and-after design. Findings revealed a reduction in length of hospital stay and a reduced waiting time for surgery from admission.

A prospective, controlled, unmatched, non-randomised study by Greenwood *et al.* (1994) to examine the effects of case management after severe head injury revealed no significant difference in physical and cognitive impairments, personality, and affective and social functioning at 6, 12, and 24 months after injury between two patient groups. Patients in the group of three case managed hospitals received normal services plus case management, while those in the control group of three hospitals received normal services. The model of case management involved patient recruitment within seven days of injury and early family contact by the case manager. A non-clinical role was adopted by the case manager. In addition to the above findings, it emerged that significantly more relatives in the case managed group reported that the accident had had a 'major' impact on the family and had disrupted their usual household routine.

Further, significantly more patients in the case managed group required supervision and care at one and two years after the injury.

Financial implications

The paucity of research investigating financial outcomes of different nursing organisational systems is noteworthy. Conflicting findings have emerged from what we have found. For example, Wilson and Dawson (1989) reported that the cost of nursing hours and medical–surgical supplies did not differ between primary and team nursing. In contrast, Gardner's (1991) longitudinal cost analysis revealed cost savings associated with primary nursing as a result of lower nurse administration costs, higher staff:patient ratios, and less use of agency nurses. Marschkle and Nolan's (1993) review of empirical work on case management revealed conflicting findings regarding the financial outcomes of case management. Empirical work cited in their review included Johnsson's (1991) research which reported a reduction in hospital expenses, and Cohen's (1991) study which found that length of stay for patients (128) post-caesarean section was reduced, although significantly more nursing hours were required in the initial hospitalisation period. In contrast, Hurley *et al.* (1989) reported no significant financial differences following the implementation of case management.

Conclusions: the way forward

This chapter has highlighted that a functional nursing system is not compatible with individualised patient care since devolved decision-making and caseload attachment are not achievable. Team nursing and primary nursing, together with case management and patient-focused care, are systems of work organisation which have the potential to facilitate the principles of individualised patient care. To realise this, however, tensions between nursing and managerial values must be reconciled. A state of equilibrium must therefore be achieved between striving to meet organisational goals and the individual needs of patients/clients. As Hewison and Wildman (1996, p. 758) assert: 'The managers of the future will need to incorporate some of the elements of nursing values into their approach'. It is argued therefore that greater devolvement of power and greater authority for nurses are required in order to enhance nurses' accountability, responsibility and autonomy, facilitating continuity of care for patients/clients and continued advancement of the nursing profession. In addition, the importance of having a supportive ward philosophy, leadership style and ward ethos in place to promote accountability, responsibility, continuity of care and good nurse–patient relationships is reiterated, together with the need for practitioners who are committed to the continued development of their knowledge and skills.

References

Adams, A. (1996) *Autonomy and influence – an examination of the concepts of nurse autonomy and influence in the context of the organisational environment of acute hospital wards.* Unpublished PhD Thesis, University of Surrey.

Audit Commission (1991) *The Virtue of Patients: Making the Best Use of Ward Nursing Resources.* HMSO, London.

Barriball, L. & While, A. (1995) The different appraisal profiles of a group of nurses and nursing aides: implications for policy initiatives. *Journal of Nursing Management*, 3, 247–54.

Batehup, L., Griffiths, P., Miller, F., Richardson, G., Spilsbury, K. & Wilson-Barnett, J. (1997) *Outcomes based evaluation of a nursing-led intermediate care unit: full project report.* By a research team from Division of Nursing & Midwifery, King's College London, and Nursing Development Unit, King's Healthcare NHS Trust, and Centre for Health Economics, University of York.

Bendall, E. (1973) *The relationship between recall and application in learning in the trainee nurse.* Unpublished PhD Thesis, University of London.

Bergen, A. (1992) Case management in the community: identifying a role for nursing. *Journal of Clinical Nursing*, 3, 251–7.

Berry, A.J. & Metcalf, C.L. (1986) Paradigms and practices; the organisation of the delivery of nursing care. *Journal of Advanced Nursing*, 11, 589–97.

Bowers, L. (1989) The significance of primary nursing. *Journal of Advanced Nursing*, 14, 13–19.

Bowman, G.S., Meddis, R. & Thompson, D.R. (1991) The development of a classification system for nurses' work methods. *International Journal of Nursing Studies*, **28**(2), 175–87.

Bradshaw, P. (1995) The recent health reforms in the United Kingdom: some tentative observations on their impact on nurses in hospital. *Journal of Advanced Nursing*, **21**(5), 975–9.

Brown, R.A. (1989) *Individualised Care: the Role of the Ward Sister.* Scutari Press, Middlesex.

Buchan, J. (1995) Are patient focused hospitals working? *Nursing Standard*, **10**(8), 30.

Burchell, H. & Jenner, E.A. (1996) The role of the nurse in patient-focused care: models of competence and implications for education and training. *International Journal of Nursing Studies*, **33**(1): 67–75.

Butterworth, T. (1994) *Working in Partnership: a Collaborative Approach to Care.* Mental Health Nursing Review, Department of Health, London.

Cavanagh, S.J. (1992) Job satisfaction of nursing staff working in hospitals. *Journal of Advanced Nursing*, 17, 704–11.

Chavasse, J. (1981) From task assignment to patient allocation: a change evaluation. *Journal of Advanced Nursing*, 6, 137–45.

Christian, S. & Norman, I.J. (1998) Clinical leadership in nursing development units. *Journal of Advanced Nursing*, **27**(1), 108–16.

Christman, N.J. (1971) Clinical performance of baccalaureate graduates. *Nursing Outlook*, **19**(1), 54–6.

Cohen, E.L. (1991) Nursing case management – does it pay? *Journal of Nursing Administration*, 21, 20–25. Cited in 'Research related to case management' (1993, P. Marschkle & M.T. Nolan), *Nursing Administration Quarterly*, **17**(3), 16–21.

Davies, S.M. (1994) An evaluation of nurse-led team care within a rehabilitation ward for elderly people. *Journal of Clinical Nursing*, 3, 25–33.

Dewing, J. (1990) Reflective practice. *Senior Nurse*, **10**(10), 26–8.

DoH (Department of Health) (1991) *The Patient's Charter*. HMSO, London.

Dowling, S., Barrett, S. & West, R. (1995) With nurse practitioners, who needs house officers? *British Medical Journal*, **311**(7000), 309–13.

Durbin, E. (1981) Comparison of Three Methods of Delivering Nursing Care. In: *The Management of Patient Care: Putting Leadership Skills to Work*, (ed. T. Kron) W.B. Saunders, Philadelphia.

Elkan, R., Hillman, R. & Robinson, J. (1995) How does P2000 affect staffing levels. *Nursing Times*, **91**(3), 11–12.

ENB (1994) *Creating Lifelong Learners – Partnerships for Care*. Guidelines for Pre-Registration Nursing Programmes of Education. English National Board for Nursing, Midwifery and Health Visiting, London.

Field, P.A. (1987) The impact of nursing theory on the clinical decision making process. *Journal of Advanced Nursing*, 12, 563–71.

Fish, D., Twinn, S. & Purr, B. (1991) *Promoting reflection: improving the supervision of practice in health visiting and initial teacher training: how to enable students to learn through professional practice*. Report No. 2. West London Institute of Higher Education, London.

Fretwell, J.E. (1980) An inquiry into the ward learning environment. Occasional Paper. *Nursing Times*, **76**(16), 69–73.

Garbett, R. (1996a) Organisation of nursing care – professional issues. *Nursing Times*, **92**(35), 9–12.

Garbett, R. (1996b) Organisation of nursing care – the role of the nurse. *Nursing Times*, **92**(34), 5–8.

Gardner, K. (1991) A summary of findings of a five-year comparison study of primary and team nursing. *Nursing Research*, **40**(2), 113–17.

Gournay, K. (1995) Mental health nurses working purposefully with people with serious and enduring mental illness – an international perspective. *International Journal of Nursing Studies*, **32**(4), 341–52.

Greenwood, R.J., McMillan, T.M., Brooks, D.N., Dunn, G., Brock, D., Dinsdale, S., Murphy, L.D. & Price, J.R. (1994) Effects of case management after severe head injury. *British Medical Journal*, **308**(6938), 1199–1205.

Hale, C. (1995) Case management and managed care. *Nursing Standard*, **9**(19), 33–5.

Harris, R., Fergusson, H. & Brooks, V. (1996) Imaginative solutions: a nursing-led unit's story. *Nursing Development News*, 16, 6–7.

Hewison, A. & Wildman, S. (1996) The theory–practice gap in nursing: a new dimension. *Journal of Advanced Nursing*, 24, 754–61.

Hospitals and Health Networks and Medicus Systems Corp. (1993) Critical Paths Survey. Evanston. Cited in 'Mapping care' (eds K. Lumsdon & M. Hagland). *Hospitals and Health Networks*, 20 October, 34–40.

Humphreys, J. (1996) Old idea, new jargon. *Nursing Standard*, **10**(52), 6.

Hunt, J.M. & Marks-Maran, D.J. (1986) *Nursing Care Plans: the Nursing Process at Work*, (2nd edn.) John Wiley & Sons, Chichester.

Hurley, R., Paul, J.E. & Freund, D. (1989) Going into gatekeeping: an empirical assessment. *Quality Review Bulletin*, 15, 306–14. Cited in 'Research related to case management,' (1993, P. Marschkle & M.T. Nolan). *Nursing Administration Quarterly*, **17**(3), 16–21.

Johnsson, J. (1991) Case study: managed care helps hospital contain costs. *Hospitals*, 65, 40–44. Cited in 'Research related to case management,' (1993, P. Marschkle & M.T. Nolan). *Nursing Administration Quarterly*, **17**(3), 16–21.

Jones, A. (1995) An analysis of case management – the efficient utility of human resources, but to what end? *Journal of Nursing Management*, 3, 143–9.

Jowett, S., Walton, I. & Payne, S. (1994) *Challenges and Change in Nurse Education: a Study of the Implementation of Project 2000*. National Foundation for Educational Research in England and Wales, Slough.

Kron, T. (ed) (1981) *The Management of Patient Care: Putting Leadership Skills to Work*. W. B. Saunders, Philadelphia.

LeClair, D. (1991) Introducing and accounting for RN case management. *Nursing Management*, **22**(3), 44-9.

Lidbetter, J. (1990) A better way to learn? *Nursing Times*, **86**(29), 61-4.

Lumsdon, K. & Hagland, M. (1993) Mapping care. *Hospitals and Health Networks*, 20 October, 34-40.

Lyon, J.C. (1993) Models of nursing care delivery and case management: clarification of terms. *Nursing Economics*, **11**(3), 163-9.

Maben, J., Latter, S., Macleod Clark, J. & Wilson-Barnett, J. (1993) The organisation of care: its influence on health education practice on acute wards. *Journal of Clinical Nursing*, 2, 355-63.

MacGuire, J., Adair, E. & Botting, D. (1993) *Primary Nursing in Elderly Care*. King's Fund Centre, London.

Marks-Maran, D. (1978) Patient allocation versus task allocation in relation to the nursing process. *Nursing Times*, 74, 413-16.

Marschkle, P. & Nolan, M.T. (1993) Research related to case management. *Nursing Administration Quarterly*, **17**(3), 16-21.

McFarlane, J.K. (1976) A charter for caring. *Journal of Advanced Nursing*, 1, 187-96.

McMahon, R. (1990) Power and collegial relations among nurses on wards adopting primary nursing and hierarchical ward management structures. *Journal of Advanced Nursing*, 15, 232-9.

Mead, D. & McGuire, J. (1993) *Innovations in Nursing Practice: the Development of Primary Nursing in Wales*. Executive Summary, NHS CYMRU, Wales.

Mills, C. (1996) The consultant nurse: a model for advanced practice. *Nursing Times*, **92**(33), 36-7.

Morgan, G. (1993) The implications of patient focused care. *Nursing Standard*, **7**(52), 37-9.

Mullen, C. (1995) *Delivering health care in a nurse-led practice development unit*. NHS Executive Value for Money Update (14), NHS Executive, Leeds.

NHSME (NHS Management Executive) (1993) *Nursing in Primary Health Care: New World, New Opportunities*. Department of Health, London.

Nazarko, L. (1998) Continuity of care for older people. *Nursing Standard*, **12**(52), 42-5.

Parasuraman, S., Drake, B.H. & Zammuto, R.F. (1982) The effect of nursing care modalities and shift assignments on nurses' work experiences and job attitudes. *Nursing Research*, **31**(6), 364-7.

Pembrey, S. (1975) From work routines to patient assignment: an experiment in ward organisation. *Nursing Times*, **71**(45), 1768-72.

Petryshen, P.R. & Petryshen, P.M. (1992) The case management model: an innovative approach to the delivery of patient care. *Journal of Advanced Nursing*, 17, 1188-94.

Phillips, T., Schostack, J., Bedford, H. & Robinson, J. (1993) *Assessment of Competencies in Nursing and Midwifery Education and Training (the ACE Project)*. Research Highlights No. 4. ENB, London.

Procter, S. (1989) The functioning of nursing routines in the management of a transient workforce. *Journal of Advanced Nursing*, 14, 180-89.

Procter, S. (1991) Patient allocation and the unqualified learner nurse. *Nursing Times*, **87**(43), 46-8.

Procter, S. (1995) Planning for continuity of carer in nursing. *Journal of Nursing Management*, 3, 169–75.

Redfern, S. (1996) Individualised patient care: its meaning and practice in a general setting. *Nursing Times Research*, **1**(1), 22–33.

Redfern, S. & Evers, H. (1995) *The Meaning and Practice of Individualised Patient Care in Nursing*. Report to the Department of Health. Nursing Research Unit, King's College London.

Redfern, S., Normand, C., Norman, I.J., Murrells, T., Christian, S., Gilmore, A., Stevens, W. & Langham, S. (1997) *External review of Department of Health-funded nursing development units*. Report to Department of Health by a team from the Nursing Research Unit, King's College, London, and the Department of Public Health & Policy, London School of Hygiene & Tropical Medicine. Nursing Research Unit, King's College, London.

Redfern, S.J. & Stevens, W. (1998) Nursing development units: their structure and orientation. *Journal of Clinical Nursing*, **7**(3), 218–26.

Reed, J. & Ground, I. (1997) *Philosophy for Nursing*. Arnold, London.

Reed, S.E. (1988) A comparison of nurse-related behaviour, philosophy of care and job satisfaction in team and primary nursing. *Journal of Advanced Nursing*, 13, 383–95.

Riches, T., Stead, L. & Espie, C. (1994) Introducing anticipated recovery pathways: a teaching hospital experience. *International Journal of Quality and Management*, 7, 21–4.

Riley, J. (1995) Fast track cardiac care. *Nursing Standard*, **9**(49), 55–6.

Salvage, J. (1985) *The Politics of Nursing*. Heinmann, London.

Salvage, J. (1990) The theory and practice of the 'new nursing'. *Nursing Times*, **86**(4), 42–5.

Saylor, C.R. (1990) Reflection and professional education: art, science and competency. *Nurse Educator*, **15**(2), 8–11.

Schön, D. (1983) *The Reflective Practitioner: How Professionals Think*. Temple Smith, London.

Sellick, K.J., Russell, S. & Beckmann, B. (1983) Primary nursing: an evaluation of its effects on patient perception of care and staff satisfaction. *International Journal of Nursing Studies*, **20**(4), 265–73.

Shamian, J. (1991) Effect of teaching decision analysis on student nurses' clinical intervention decision making. *Research in Nursing and Health*, 14, 59–66.

Shiell, A., Kenny, P. & Farnworth, M.G. (1993) The role of the clinical nurse co-ordinator in the provision of cost-effective orthopaedic services for elderly people. *Journal of Advanced Nursing*, 18, 1424–8.

Slater, D. (1967) *The Slater Nursing Competencies Rating Scale*. College of Nursing, Wayne State University, Detroit.

Smith, P. (1991) The nursing process: raising the profile of emotional care in nurse training. *Journal of Advanced Nursing*, 16, 74–81.

Smith, P.A. (1992) *The Emotional Labour of Nursing: Its Impact on Interpersonal Relations, Management and the Educational Environment in Nursing*. Macmillan Education Ltd, London.

Tahan, H. (1993) The nurse case manager in acute care settings. *Journal of Nursing Administration*, 23, 53–61.

Thomas, L.H. (1992) Qualified nurse and nursing auxiliary perceptions of their work environment in primary, team and functional nursing wards. *Journal of Advanced Nursing*, 17, 373–82.

Thomas, L.H. (1993) Comparing qualified nurse and auxiliary roles. *Nursing Times*, **89**(38), 45–8.

Thomas, L.H. (1994) A comparison of the verbal interactions of qualified nurses and nursing auxiliaries in primary, team and functional nursing wards. *International Journal of Nursing Studies*, **31**(3), 231–44.

Thomas, L.H. & Bond, S. (1990) Towards defining the organisation of nursing care in hospital wards: an empirical study. *Journal of Advanced Nursing*, 15, 1106–12.

Thomas, L.H., McColl, E., Priest, J. & Bond, S. (1996) The impact of primary nursing on patient satisfaction. *Nursing Times*, **92**(22), 36–8.

UKCC (1992a) *Code of Professional Conduct for the Nurse, Midwife and Health Visitor* (2nd edn). United Kingdom Central Council for Nursing, Midwifery and Health Visiting, London.

UKCC (1992b) *The Scope of Professional Practice*. United Kingdom Central Council for Nursing, Midwifery and Health Visiting, London.

Vlerick, P. (1996) Burnout and work organisation in hospital wards: a cross-validation study. *Work and Stress*, **10**(3), 257–65.

Wallace, M. & Gough, P. (1995) The UKCC's criteria for specialist and advanced nursing practice. *British Journal of Nursing*, **4**(16), 939–44.

Waterman, H., Waters, K. & Awenat, Y. (1996) The introduction of case management on a rehabilitation floor. *Journal of Advanced Nursing*, 24, 960–67.

Webb, C. & Pontin, D. (1996) Introducing primary nursing: nurses' opinions. *Journal of Clinical Nursing*, 5, 351–8.

White, E., Riley, E., Davies, S. & Twinn, S. (1994) *A Detailed Study of the Relationship between Teaching, Support, Supervision and Role Modelling in Clinical Areas within the Context of P2000 Courses*. ENB, London.

Wilson, N.M. & Dawson, P. (1989) A comparison of primary nursing and team nursing in a geriatric long-term care setting. *International Journal of Nursing Studies*, **26**(1), 1–13.

Wilson-Barnett, J., Butterworth, T., White, E., Twinn, S., Davies, S. & Riley, L. (1995) Clinical support and the Project 2000 nursing student: factors influencing this process. *Journal of Advanced Nursing*, 21, 1152–8.

7 Education for Nursing: Preparation for Professional Practice

Julia Roberts and K. Louise Barriball

Nurse education has been the subject of widespread debate and controversy for several decades (e.g. RCN 1942, MoH 1947, RCN/NCN 1964, DHSS 1972, UKCC 1986, UKCC 1994). In the UK a particular focus for debate has been the educational preparation of nurses prior to registration. Concerns have been raised about the adequacy of the apprenticeship model of preparation, that is the Registered General Nurse (RGN) programme (and similar programmes for mental nurses (RMN) and learning disability nurses (RNMH)) in fulfilling students' educational requirements since the 1940s (Ramprogus 1995). In addition to educational factors, the search for a different approach to the preparation of nurses on pre-registration nurse education programmes was stimulated also by student and teacher dissatisfaction with the RGN practice-based model of nurse preparation (French 1989) and growing concerns about recruitment and retention (GNC 1969, Telford 1979). In addition, new demands and expectations of professional practice in the light of changing health care needs, as well as developments in the delivery of health care services, have had significant implications for the role of nurses which needed to be reflected in pre-registration nurse education programmes in order to ensure fitness for purpose (RCN/NCN 1985, UKCC 1986).

Pressure to review the educational and professional development of UK nurses arose therefore for several reasons. Demographic and epidemiological trends over the last two decades have impinged on health care provision, which in turn has posed significant challenges for nurse education. Specific changes in health care needs have included:

- An increase in the level of preventable mortality (Smith & Jacobsen 1988)
- Increasing levels of chronic illness (OPCS 1989)
- An increase in the elderly population (OPCS 1987)
- Acute health care increasingly involving only short episodic stays in hospital (Audit Commission 1986)
- A focus on primary care as well as a shift towards care in the community (NHS & Community Care Act 1990).

Equally significant have been technological advances throughout the health care field with the need for requisite technological skills among health care personnel. Further, the increased emphasis on evidence-based care (Davidoff *et al*. 1995, Deighan & Hitch 1995, Batstone & Edwards 1996) has meant that the concept of a 'knowledgeable doer' has assumed increased importance and the need to further develop the research base on which nursing practice ought to rely has received added impetus. Educational reform in the shape of the Project 2000/Diploma of Higher Education (DipHE) programme was viewed as a means of meeting such needs. Indeed, the UKCC (1986) promoted the value of the programme by arguing that each student would leave the course 'a thinking person with analytical skills' (p. 4) able to function effectively in a changing health care environment.

The intervening decade also witnessed increasing concerns regarding registered nurses' skills post-registration, resulting in legislative action by the profession's statutory body (UKCC 1994). The Council's standards for education following registration, commonly known as PREP (UKCC 1994), set out new regulations for ensuring that all registered nurses remain responsive to changing health care needs and practice throughout their professional careers. The document argued that this would be achieved by linking periodic registration (i.e. every three years) with evidence of continued professional development (e.g. through the use of professional portfolios) and learning (i.e. a minimum of five days of study in three years) as well as providing standards for practice and education beyond initial registration (e.g. specialist practice). The impact of PREP both on nursing in general and individual practitioners remains uncertain since its introduction has been very recent. Central to the developments in both pre- and post-registration education, however, has been the debate regarding the academic and skills base of nurse education.

The latter debate is the focus of this chapter. Key developments in both pre- and post-registration nurse education in the UK are discussed, beginning with the demise of the apprenticeship model of preparation, the development of undergraduate degree programmes and the inception of the DipHE programme. The chapter turns then to an analysis of key issues in post-registration education, and discussion of recent trends in the management of nurse education. We conclude by setting out the background to occupational standards and competency-based education and describe the development of National Vocational Qualifications (NVQs) to higher levels. What emerges from this is an increasingly blurred distinction between academic, vocational and professional education. Although the focus is on education developments in the UK the issues raised are those which are relevant to nurse education world-wide.

Academic versus skills-based curricula

Professional nurse education has moved away from the earlier apprenticeship style model of pre-registration programmes towards curricula which have an increased focus on knowledge acquisition. It is interesting, however, that other areas of professional preparation such as teacher training have moved once more towards a practice-based curriculum in an attempt to reduce the theory–practice gap and enhance the acquisition of requisite skills (Maguire 1994, Jowett 1995). The introduction of the DipHE programme heralded, however, the end of the practice-based model of pre-registration nurse education.

The apprenticeship model: a practice base

The Registered General Nurse (RGN) programme was based on an apprentice-type model. The model had as its focus the learning of a craft or skill on site (i.e. the clinical practice environment) under the guidance of a skilled supervisor (Beckett 1984). The Lancet Commission (1932) summarised the profession's early view of the system when they suggested that:

> 'The element of apprenticeship is regarded by most of the leaders of the nursing profession, at least in this country, as a far more important part of a nurse's training than her theoretical studies.'

(p. 28 para. 34)

The result was a training system based primarily on experience gained in the clinical setting as a means of acquiring knowledge and skills. The courses were designed around periods of clinical experience with blocks of theory in a health service education setting focusing on hospital-based care (UKCC 1980, p. 12). In view of the volume of material to be covered within a limited time span (between 24 and 28 weeks in total were devoted to teaching – GNC Circular 69/4/3) and the authoritarian style pervading schools of nursing, traditional didactic teaching strategies were employed which followed closely the medical education model.

Underpinning the learning experience was a major service contribution, with student nurses providing 75% of all bedside nursing care (DHSS 1972, Moores & Moult 1979). Indeed, students in training made up 20% of nursing and midwifery staff in hospitals and were integral to effective service delivery (UKCC 1986). The combination of theoretical periods with associated practical experience had much to commend it. Alexander (1983) has pointed to the potential for the integration of theory and practice, for example in the use of the nursing process. However, the apprenticeship model posed a number of dilemmas. Chapman (1980) has highlighted the conflict posed by joint student/employee status leading to situations in which, due to the pressure of work, students became fixated by task performance with neither the time nor the inclination to consider the why or wherefore of the situation. The reality of service allocation in many instances, therefore, may have thwarted educational endeavour. Furthermore, a training model cannot be dissociated from the wider social and economic context or the institutional framework in which it occurs (Edwards *et al.* 1993) and the RGN model proved particularly vulnerable to problems within the institutional setting.

The adequacy of the model with its assumption that trained nurses would teach and supervise student nurses was increasingly questioned (Fretwell 1980, 1985, Orton 1981, Reid 1985, Jacka & Lewin 1987). Fretwell's (1980) early study highlighted the key role played by the ward sister in creating a positive learning environment, as well as the lack of formal preparation to fulfil such a role. Equally the relationship between increased clinical workload and reduced clinical teaching emerged as a key issue. A later study by Reid (1985) examined the training capacity of clinical areas. Reid's findings again highlighted the significant role played by the ward sister in determining the quality of the clinical learning environment as well as the limited teaching actually received by students in practice, in particular from clinical teachers. Such findings posed questions regarding the adequacy of support received by traditionally trained students in clinical practice.

A further criticism of the apprenticeship model related to its industrial rather than professional focus, specifically its emphasis on psychomotor skills acquisition and task-centred approach (Fretwell 1980, French 1989). Indeed, it has been argued that the repetition of tasks may inhibit the individual's capacity for wider knowledge and professional development (Fretwell 1983, Melia 1987, Fish *et al.* 1991) and that an emphasis on the performance of activities with little time for reflection may undermine the potential for learning (Chapman 1980, Orton 1981, Ogier 1982, UKCC 1986, Greenwood 1993). Concerns therefore regarding the efficacy of the model were expressed repeatedly by nurses' official bodies (UKCC 1982, 1985, 1988, RCN/NCN 1985, ENB 1989) and formed the backdrop to the introduction of the DipHE programme (UKCC 1986). Prior to the introduction of the DipHE programme, though, nursing degree programmes offered an alternative to the apprenticeship model and provided the academic base of nursing.

Nursing degree programmes: an academic base

Nursing degree programmes, based within institutions of higher education, are education-led with students having supernumerary status during their clinical placements. Unlike the USA where the first nursing degree programme was established as early as 1909 at the University of Minnesota (Logan 1987), the first pioneering degree programmes in Britain were only established in the 1950s. Although it was suggested at the time that nursing could only benefit from links with higher education (Carter 1956), these links were slow to develop. Fitzpatrick *et al.* (1993) have argued that this was, in part, due to a reluctance to accept the potential value of a highly educated nurse whose principles of practice were derived from a knowledge of research. However, despite this initial hesitancy a number of degree programmes were established subsequently throughout the country. Such initiatives were in part a response to continued calls for reform in nurse education (RCN/NCN 1964, DHSS 1972).

Each degree programme is unique and embedded within its own history within higher education (Phillips *et al.* 1993). But all are required to fulfil two key criteria: to operate at an acceptable academic level, and to incorporate sufficient clinical experience to enable students to qualify as clinically competent and enter the relevant part of the professional nurses' register. Nursing degree courses have been usually of four years' duration, although recently a number of three year degree courses have been validated (ENB 1991). Jones (1996) has suggested that the goals of level 3 curricula independent of subject domain include aspects of cognitive learning (rationality, intellectual perspective, creativity and intellectual integrity) which relate overall to the development of cognitive abilities. Nurse education at this level therefore is concerned with the development of cognitive skills and their application to practice and, within the context of degree programmes, aims to focus on the development of thinking and questioning skills as well as a commitment to self-directed and life-long learning (Collins 1984, Atkins & Williams 1995). These key outcomes have been echoed in the DipHE programme (UKCC 1986).

DipHE programme: a theoretical base

The DipHE programme was inaugurated with Statutory Instrument No. 1456 (1989) and has now replaced the RGN model of nurse education. The diploma curricula were designed expressly to redress the recognised inadequacies of the RGN programmes and were therefore education-led and involved a service contribution of only 20% during the course. It was anticipated that this innovation would help solve the problem of poor retention rates on pre-registration nurse education programmes (Dean 1987) and facilitate improved recruitment rates in the light of demographic trends (OPCS 1994).

A fundamental change with the inception of the DipHE programme related to its academic level and subsequent course content. Nursing's statutory body, the UKCC, stated that the diplomate would be:

'A knowledgeable doer, able to marshal information, to make an assessment of need, devise a plan of care and implement, monitor and evaluate it.'

(UKCC 1986, p. 5)

The intended outcome was to produce a critical, autonomous professional, able to respond flexibly to different situations and capable of problem solving and addressing complex issues (UKCC 1986, Miller *et al.* 1994, Jinks 1994). A further change has been the major shift in emphasis away from the medical model towards a health-normality paradigm (Robinson 1991a). The focus of the new programme was on holistic, individualised care with an equal emphasis on both community and institutional settings (UKCC, 1986). Despite these ambitions, however, there have been significant problems associated with the introduction of the diploma model of nurse preparation.

A number of nurse teachers had not taught at diploma level before the introduction of the new RN programme and were unsure of the academic level required (White *et al.* 1994). Furthermore, the new diploma programme aimed at producing a 'thinking' practitioner (UKCC 1986) which necessitated the development of reflective skills (Schön 1983, Akinsanya 1990, Miller *et al.* 1994). Self-directed learning has been shown to improve the quality of learning and increase student motivation as well as providing an appropriate teaching strategy for adult learners (Jones 1981, Knowles 1990). The growth of reflection through self-directed study, small group work and individual tutorials has, however, posed difficulties in that the large cohort sizes and restricted physical environment in some areas has mitigated against effective student facilitation (Elkan *et al.* 1993, Jowett *et al.* 1994, Luker *et al.* 1995). Indeed, Payne *et al.* (1991), in a study of the six demonstration districts which introduced the DipHE programme, found that many teachers reported reverting to 'talk and chalk' teaching methods when confronted with such large student numbers. In other instances, there are examples of teachers favouring a 'teach-yourself' approach (Burnard & Morrisson 1991).

The expectation that the qualifications of students entering diploma programmes would be higher has also been confounded. The reverse has proved to be the case, which is consistent with the UKCC's (1987) target for widening the entry gate into nursing. The raised academic level of the new RN programme (equivalent to CNAA CATS at 120 points at level I and 120 points at level II) is therefore not without its difficulties with the mixed abilities of some intakes, ranging from DC (Dennis Child) test candidates to graduates, posing problems for teachers and students alike (Jowett *et al.* 1992a,b, Elkan *et al.* 1993, 1995, Houltram 1996). Houltram (1996) explored the relationship between entry age, entry qualifications and academic performance among three intakes of a DipHE programme using a retrospective analysis of academic results. He found that younger candidates (17–21 years) recruited via the DC test route performed the least well and had the lowest overall mean scores coupled with a high discontinuation rate. In view of this, he questioned the wisdom of a broad entry gate and suggested that if it was to continue, the mechanisms for student support would need to be strengthened. Although not readily generalisable, these findings are of interest in view of the recruitment difficulties experienced by a number of institutions (Waters 1996).

Unlike the RGN students who were health service employees, DipHE students have full student status with the exception of a period of rostered service towards the end of the course. Elkan (1995) reviewing the literature on the DipHE programme concluded that there was widespread support for the concept of supernumerary status. However, Elkan *et al.* (1993), in the second phase of an evaluative study of one of the six demonstration districts, suggested a lack of clarity regarding the concept of supernumerary status coupled with poor operationalisation in practice. Indeed, Payne *et al.* (1991) have suggested that full student status means that nurse education is now, more than in the past, dependent on the goodwill of service staff for the provision of high quality clinical learning environments.

This level of dependency on the goodwill of service staff is compounded by the apparent lack of knowledge that clinical staff have regarding the nature of the diploma programme (Robinson 1992). However, the problems of learning in the clinical environment are not unique to the DipHE programme, but are resonant of the continued problem of how best to facilitate learning and integrate theory and practice (Sloan & Slevin 1991). Evidence suggests that the supervision of students deteriorates with poor staffing levels (Jowett *et al.* 1992a). Indeed, White *et al.*'s (1994) qualitative study of mentorship and supervision of diploma students found that learning opportunities were reduced due to competing demands on practitioners' time as well as confusion regarding the concept and operationalisation of mentorship programmes. In addition, the task of appropriate supervision and teaching may be confounded in some areas by extended shift patterns, as witnessed by Reid *et al.* (1991) in a study of educational activities on wards operating a 12-hour shift system.

The higher education context

The introduction of the DipHE programme was accompanied by the recommendation that schools of nursing forge links with institutions of higher education (ENB 1989). Subsequent institutional mergers have resulted in extended periods of upheaval (Kenrick 1993). Akinsanya (1990) depicted the current trend as an attempt to move away from the 'mono-technique' school of nursing into an environment where students are able to interact with other disciplines. The pace of this change, however, has been unprecedented (Lathlean 1989, Jowett *et al.* 1994). The subsequent effects of changes in educational structure, ethos and culture on staff morale and in turn on the student body, cannot be underestimated and it will take a considerable time before equilibrium is restored (Miles *et al.* 1988, Thomason 1988, Rosenholtz 1989). The implications of such changes for the role and function of the nurse teacher have been particularly significant (Luker *et al.* 1995).

The inauguration of the DipHE programme coupled with subsequent mergers with institutions of higher education has led to high levels of reported stress among nurse teachers (Payne *et al.* 1991, Robinson 1991a, Elkan & Robinson 1993). Robinson (1991b), in an evaluative study of the implementation of the new programme in one college, suggested high levels of stress due to role confusion, lack of direction and overall uncertainty. Other studies have indicated problems associated with conflicting demands on nurse teachers' time (Payne *et al.* 1991, Elkan & Robinson 1993, White *et al.* 1994) and lack of preparation for the new role (Clifford 1995, Luker *et al.* 1995). Increased stress has resulted also from the expectation that all nurse teachers will achieve graduate status (DoH 1989), a pressure which was exacerbated by the new mergers with higher education institutions and the subsequent need to attain academic credibility leading to a rush to obtain graduate status, especially higher degrees (Payne *et al.* 1991, Luker *et al.* 1995).

A further source of conflict for nurse teachers during this period has been the pressure to maintain clinical competence (DoH 1989, Clifford 1995) and engage in a teaching/facilitating role within the clinical area (White *et al.* 1994). Crotty and Butterworth's (1992) literature review on the emerging role of nurse teachers in diploma programmes suggested that the majority of the teachers' time was spent in classroom teaching and administration. Indeed, the evidence suggested that few nurse teachers engaged in clinical practice regularly and that, in the main, their role in the clinical area was of a purely liaison nature (Payne *et al.* 1991, Luker *et al.* 1995). White *et al.* (1994) had similar findings and highlighted the implications for the level of teaching and supervision provided for the large numbers of diploma students placed in the clinical area at any one time; findings which echo the difficulties encountered by students on the RGN model of pre-registration nurse education during their clinical placements (Fretwell 1980, Reid 1985, Jacka & Lewin 1987).

It was anticipated that the new programme delivered in conjunction with institutions of higher education would prove more attractive to potential recruits than the old RGN model of pre-registration education. Jowett (1995) has highlighted, however, the inherent contradiction which currently exists in that while the diploma programme is underpinned by a theoretical base and is delivered in partnership with institutions of higher education, the degree of input from the latter remains variable. There is a potential conflict between liberal views regarding the aims of higher education including personal and cultural development, and an increasing emphasis on the development of specific vocational skills.

Clinical skills: fitness for purpose

Research suggests that students on DipHE programmes experience stress when in the clinical area due to a perceived lack of skills (White *et al.* 1994, Hamill 1995). Indeed, the curriculum content has been criticised by diplomates for a lack of focus on the development of clinical skills. Students in Macleod-Clark *et al.*'s (1996) exploratory study of diplomates' perceptions of the philosophy and practice of nursing identified a perceived lack of practical skills as a shortcoming of the diploma programme. Diploma students in While *et al.*'s (1995) comparative study of the outcomes of pre-registration nurse education programmes expressed similar concerns. Furthermore, concern has been raised by clinical staff regarding the lack of clinical exposure for students during the common foundation programme (Robinson 1992).

Criticism has also been voiced by nurse managers that current pre-registration nurse education programmes lack a well defined skills base (Carlisle *et al.* 1996). Such criticisms are not unique to nursing but reflect a perceived skills deficit within the British workforce in general when compared with our European competitors (Keep 1993, Kemp & Seagraves 1995). The internal market of the NHS, introduced by the NHS and Community Care Act 1990, has enabled provider units to exercise greater freedom in employment practices coupled with the ability to determine the requisite skill mix. Whether this will change with the policies of the Labour administration is, as yet, unclear. Carlisle *et al.* (1996), in an extensive study of the fitness for purpose of the DipHE programme education reforms, highlighted some of the widespread concerns among senior nurse managers regarding 'basic' skills acquisition among diplomates.

The DipHE programme was inaugurated in response to a number of factors, including: repeated criticisms that educational standards were compromised by the employee status of student nurses and their obligation to fulfil service/manpower needs (Bell 1983, Reid 1985); the realisation that the health care sector like other employers was faced with the difficulty of meeting recruitment and manpower targets with the fall in the birth rate between the years 1964–1979 (OPCS 1987); and to help prepare nurses to deliver care in the new health care environment of the year 2000 and beyond (UKCC 1986). It is noteworthy, therefore, that disquiet exists about how successful the DipHE programme has been in addressing these issues.

The DipHE programme is based on the premise that the qualified nurse of the future will have moved away from direct care delivery towards a more managerial/supervisory role. The nature of the changing occupational roles within the health service, in particular the introduction of the new health care worker and the programme of preparation which they undertake (National Vocational Qualification), have indeed led to a redistribution of responsibilities among nurses in both community and institutional settings with health care assistants increasingly taking over 'core' nursing tasks (Carlisle *et al.* 1996). However, the call for nurses to assume certain activities previously performed by junior doctors and to develop their scope of practice (UKCC 1992a, Greenhalgh 1994) has raised the level and range of clinical skills increasingly demanded of nurses and reinforces the significance of the perceived lack of 'basic' skills currently acquired by nurses during their initial educational preparation into the profession.

Education following registration

The Platt Report (RCN/NCN 1964) argued that the pattern of post-basic nursing education needed changing in the light of the demands made by new basic nursing education. Thirty years later, following consultation with members of the profession, the UKCC (1994) set out its standards for education and practice for registered nurses to complement the DipHE programme. Integral to these standards is the provision of a systematic framework of professional development for all registered nurses reflective of their roles in the delivery of health care.

During the 1980s there was growing concern within the profession that some nurses did not update their knowledge or develop their skills following registration (Myco 1980, Barnett 1981, O'Brien & Heyman 1989, Chiarella 1990) and there was increasing evidence that much of the continuing professional development activity of nurses was ad hoc and inequitable (Studdy & Hunt 1980, Lathlean & Farnish 1984, Rogers 1987, Clarke & Rees 1989, Mackereth 1989). In addition, consideration of how the role of the nurse should develop and progress in order to meet new demands within the health service stimulated interest in the importance of appropriate post-registration or continuing professional education in nursing (DoH 1994, ENB 1994, UKCC 1994). In particular, the educational preparation undertaken by nurses with new roles and responsibilities such as clinical nurse specialists, nurse practitioners and advanced nurse practitioners has attracted increasing attention (David 1994, Dowling *et al.* 1995, Wilson-Barnett 1995, Wright 1995).

The development of professional practice following registration

Continued development of the nurse's role has been sustained by the potential for new patterns of working and delivering health care to patients created by the purchaser–provider split and a shift in emphasis from secondary to primary care (NHS & Community Care Act 1990). Other important factors include a reduction in the hours worked by junior doctors (DoH 1991) and an increasing focus on health promotion and disease prevention (DoH 1992) as well as demands for effective use of human resources in the health service (Carr-Hill *et al.* 1992).

Adjustments to nurses' roles have predominately followed an inherently task orientated approach re-emphasising the academic versus skills base debate which has dominated discussions about pre-registration nurse preparation for many years. While there have been schemes where individual nurses have focused on the provision of individualised and holistic care for patients, often with specific disorders such as diabetes or Parkinson's disease, changes to nurses' roles typically follow a highly medical model of practice with nurses undertaking some of the responsibilities traditionally performed by doctors, for example, venepuncture and cannulation, Doppler assessment and some minor surgery and other specialised procedures such as endoscopies.

There is some demonstrable evidence of the value to patients and clients as well as the service of nurses extending and expanding their practice, such as greater patient satisfaction and accessibility, increased continuity of care and a reduction in the hours worked by junior doctors (Hamilton 1993, Hammond *et al.* 1995, Marsh & Dawes 1995, Touche Ross 1995, Rees & Kinnersley 1996). Opportunities for developing new skills and retraining in different specialist fields may also be important factors in encouraging nurses to return to practice (OPCS 1991). Perhaps more important than this evidence, however, is the considerable optimism which exists regarding the impact new roles for nurses will have on the provision of services. Dunn (1997), for example, argues that:

'What was needed in the past, and is still needed, is a focus on how the health care system can best be designed to provide high quality care to all at an affordable price ... The role of the advanced nurse practitioner should increase the likelihood of this taking place.'

(p. 818)

While such claims may be unfounded at present, it is belief in this type of potential which has sustained the enormous and almost unchecked growth in the scope of nurses' roles in recent years.

Adjustments to the scope of professional practice and the emergence of new roles for nurses, however, are not without controversy and have encountered opposition. Concerns have been raised, for example, about the lack of comparative data on the effectiveness of these roles and the absence of cost benefit analyses (Watson *et al.* 1994, Wilson-Barnett & Beech 1994, Centre for Health Economics 1995) and how extensions to professional practice are monitored (Denner 1995). There are also debates about what skills and responsibilities it is appropriate for nurses to undertake (Vaughan 1989, Hoover & van Ooijen 1995) with Sutton and Smith (1995) calling for nurses to develop their roles in directions other than taking on discarded medical tasks. Nemes (1994) questions whether increasing specialisation improves the care given to patients and suggests that the driving force behind such changes is based not on the needs of patients but rather on the needs of medicine. In addition, the impact that increasing specialisation may have on the value of generalist or core skills traditionally associated with nursing remains unclear (Wade & Moyer 1989, Dowling *et al.* 1995).

While Trnobranski (1994) has argued that expansion and extension offers career advancement for nurses wishing to remain in clinical practice, others have questioned the level of job satisfaction and career progress experienced by nurses in new roles (David 1994, Wilson-Barnett 1995). Wilson-Barnett (1995), for example, has noted that specialist practice in particular may become repetitive, leaving nurses frustrated and feeling blocked in their careers. Concerns have also been raised about the uncertainties which surround the educational preparation of nurses increasing the scope of their practice (Jordan 1993, David 1994, Gillan 1995). This uncertainty has arisen for a number of reasons.

Education and practice following registration: the uncertainties

There is little agreement in the definitions of the roles of clinical nurse specialists, nurse practitioners or advanced nurse practitioners or to what extent their roles and functions differ or overlap. There is also a lack of clarity in defining many new roles in nursing in terms of degree of autonomy and accountability and level of practice. Without a definition of the core concepts underpinning different posts it is difficult for education providers to develop appropriate course curricula and, in particular, make decisions about how specialist or generalist the content of courses should be and whether or not there ought to be core subjects included in curricula.

Nursing titles such as clinical nurse specialist, nurse practitioner and advanced nurse practitioner have historically been applied to posts without being associated with specific criteria, grades or educational qualifications. This has led to confusion which has resulted in enormous variation in the length, structure, level and content of courses available to nurses developing their roles (Coopers & Lybrand 1995, Dowling *et al.* 1995, Bellone 1996, Higgins 1997). There are also a number of reports of nurses undertaking new roles without any formal training (Marsh & Dawes 1995, Rees & Kinnersley 1996). Indeed, Wilson-Barnett (1995) has noted that training 'on the job' often typifies the mode of preparation of many nurses undertaking new roles following registration.

Appropriate educational preparation, however, is important for a number of reasons: to provide a service which is underpinned by a sound knowledge and skills base (DoH 1994); to enable nurses to determine their repertoire of skills and thus which tasks they are competent to undertake to support safe practice (Lawson & Emmerson 1995, Wright 1995, Rees & Kinnersley 1996); and to ensure that nurses recognise the legal and professional issues surrounding their practice. Preparation for practice must also ensure that service requirements for a skilled and educated nursing workforce are met (NHS Executive 1996) as well as professional and academic requirements for approval and recognition (UKCC 1992bc).

PREP (UKCC 1994) was introduced to give nurses the opportunity to pursue continuing professional development activities throughout their careers, to meet their changing professional and personal needs as well as the needs of the service within a systematic framework. It was hoped this would avoid the fragmentation created by divisions between in-service and post-registration education which has traditionally typified the provision of continuing professional education for nurses in the UK. To achieve this, however, the profession needed to legislate for standards of practice which would require employers to define roles and responsibilities within these standards.

New standards for educational preparation

The UKCC (1994) published standards for the education and practice of the specialist practitioner and the English National Board for Nursing, Midwifery and Health Visiting (ENB 1994) issued guidelines for educational programmes leading to the qualification of specialist practitioner with which all courses had to comply for approval by 1998. It is anticipated that specialist practitioners will be prepared to degree level reflecting the trend in pre-registration nurse preparation of forging strong links with institutions of higher education and raising the academic base of nursing. There remains, however, confusion regarding how the role of the nurse practitioner fits in with the standards for specialist practice and educational preparation outlined in PREP (Pearson *et al.* 1995). In addition, the UKCC will not be issuing standards for the practice and education for advanced practice because it is unclear to what extent this level of practice meets the following criteria:

(1) Responsiveness to patient or client need
(2) Appropriateness to all care settings (i.e. its universal application)
(3) Durability to sustain practice through continuing changes in the delivery of health care.

The impact this decision will have on both the practice and educational activities of nurses using or intending to use the title of advanced nurse practitioner is unclear. A further consultation process exploring standards for a higher level of practice is in progress (UKCC 1998). However, the trend towards master's level degree programmes for nurses pursuing a clinical career is likely to continue.

These courses have been developed partly to meet the growing demand among nurses for advanced education but primarily to meet the requirements of local trusts for advancing the technical skills of their nursing personnel in particular clinical or priority areas (e.g. West Midlands RHA 1995); for example, neonatal intensive care, accident and emergency, midwifery, obstetric and critical care as well as paediatrics. As these courses are relatively new, little evaluation has so far taken place although a number of evaluation projects are underway. Consequently, the appropriateness of this level of education to underpin practice and competencies, as well as how effectively the development of advanced cognitive skills will combine with the acquisition and application of advanced psycho motor skills in the practice setting, remains unclear. Of particular interest will be the extent to which master's level preparation enhances nurses' roles and the level of interplay between the changing scope of practice and advanced academic preparation.

In the absence of a national framework or standards for advanced practice and, until recently, specialist practice, the service has largely taken the lead in directing and managing the preparation for practice beyond registration (Gillan 1995). This has meant that both education and practice initiatives have tended to focus on meeting local and organisationally generated needs and have followed an almost exclusively medical model of care. These trends may not sit comfortably with the profession's ambitions for autonomous and holistic practice and may frustrate those advocating that nurses reappraise the impact of taking on increasing numbers of technical tasks both to the practice of nursing and patient care (e.g. Nemes 1994, Sutton & Smith 1995). This, coupled with the profession's focus on individual accountability to underpin the changing scope of nursing practice (UKCC 1992a), means that there is enormous potential for conflict (Land *et al.* 1996).

The development of nursing practice requires flexibility to ensure that nurses remain responsive to changing health care needs and this flexibility needs to be reflected in nurse education. On the basis of pragmatic considerations, it may be that service dominance in the development of education opportunities for nurses following registration is the most effective way of ensuring this. This development undermines, however, the ambitions of the reforms at both pre- and post-registration vis-a-vis the profession's management of nurse education.

The management of nurse education

The demise of the old apprenticeship style model of nurse preparation with its close links to practice was seen as the end of service-driven nurse education, and the establishment of links between nursing and institutions of higher education was heralded as a further step away from an apprenticeship curriculum model. Indeed, Witz (1994) has commented that the introduction of the DipHE programme represented a bid to create nurse control over nurse education by: 'enabling greater control by nurses over what is taught, how it is taught and, crucially, where it is taught' (p. 28). The reality, however, has proved somewhat different. The introduction of the purchaser–provider split and the advent of educational contracting means in essence an increase in the power of service to determine the future shape of nurse education.

In 1995 the NHS Executive published details of a new framework for planning and commissioning education and training, a central element of which was education consortia (Humphreys 1996a). Education consortia consist of representatives from health care provider organisations and purchasing authorities who in due course will take on responsibility for commissioning non-medical education and training (NMET). In 1996 there were 45 consortia in the UK (Weight 1996). This innovation has led to the development of competitive training environments in which neither regions or trusts will be interested in established historical relationships or boundaries (Humphreys 1995). What has been created in effect is a complex 'quasi-market' economy in which colleges compete for clients (Le Grand & Bartlett 1992, Humphreys 1996a,b). In such circumstances, the survival of colleges will be dependent on effective management and the requisite attitudes and skills of staff (Humphreys 1996b). The extent to which this scenario will change under the more collaborative and less competitive relationship between NHS trusts advocated by the new Labour government is, as yet, uncertain.

Roques (1996) points to the change in educational culture which is emerging as educational institutions have to come to terms with both a customer focus and a market culture, neither of which necessarily fits with the notion of academic freedom. Courses can no longer be determined by educational criteria alone with little adaptation for constantly changing needs in clinical practice. The purpose of consortia is to purchase the education that they need and it is they who will determine the type and content of courses (Stanwick 1994). A shift in thinking is therefore required from education providers to ensure that they comply with the purchasing agendas of consortia, who will want evidence of the resource implications, cost-effectiveness and fitness for purpose of different educational offerings.

With regards to continuing professional education in particular, marketing success is likely to accompany programmes which offer flexibility in the management of courses to avoid the duplication of learning, variability in the topics which students can choose to undertake to meet their specific learning needs and the acquisition and assessment of highly technical skills to meet service requirements for increasing specialisation. Consequently education providers have had to become far more proactive and responsive to service needs, rather than designing and delivering programmes determined solely by the educational institution. Dilemmas exist with the pressure to respond to customer requirements, even if viewed as academically unsound, because as Stanwick (1994) points out, educational institutions which fail to deliver the goods demanded by the customer will lose out to those education providers that rise to the challenge.

It may be argued therefore that the power of service vis-a-vis nurse education has never been greater. Education consortia perceive their needs in terms of specific clinical skills and psycho-motor competencies. Such needs by their very nature are reductionist and are potentially at odds with the ethos of higher education as a provider of a broad educational experience. The economic power of educational consortia, however, means that they rather than educators have the potential to shape the nature of future nurse education curricula.

Higher National Vocational Qualifications (NVQs)

In this chapter we have focused up to now on the development of education for professional nurses at pre- and post-registration level. In this section we turn to consider the development of vocational qualifications that has taken place in parallel with nurse education reforms. NVQs have now been extended to include the health and social care professions and are likely to exert a major influence on the future of professional nurse education.

Occupational standards and their origins

The origins of what are known as occupational standards can be traced to functional analysis of tasks based on structured observation that developed mainly in North America. The outcome of this became known as competence-based education that was widely used in initial teacher training in the USA in the 1980s (Eraut 1994).

Functional analysis methodology was developed by McMahon and Carter (1990) who analysed jobs and their component parts functionally (stage one) and then identified the skills required to undertake the job (stage two). Functional analysis remains today the process through which occupational standards are developed for health and social care. However, structured observation has been replaced largely by techniques that seek consensus through consultation. A widely used procedure is to bring together in workshops service-users, employers and employees and ask them to describe the functions of particular work roles (tasks involved, skills required, and the range of settings within which these tasks are performed) and to agree best practice for performance of these functions (Care Sector Consortium 1997). The outcome is a set of draft standards in the form of units of competence. These units comprise elements with associated performance criteria underpinning knowledge and range statements. Draft standards are circulated widely for consultation and modified in the light of feedback received.

In the UK the growth of competence-based education was driven by concerns about the low skills of the workforce, which were perceived as one cause of the country's limited competitiveness in world markets (Mitchell & Cuthbert 1989). The Review of Educational Qualifications (Manpower Services Commission and Department for Education and Science 1986) pointed to the need for a framework for Scottish and National Vocational Qualifications (S/NVQ) and led to the National Council for Vocational Qualifications (NCVQ) being established in 1986. But in so doing the review adopted a relatively narrow task-centred definition of competence as 'the ability to perform satisfactorily an occupation or range of occupational tasks'. This limited definition of competence and its outcomes – long lists of standards – meant that national occupational standards, S/NVQs and competence-based education were seen as completely unsuitable for the education and training of the professions. Thus, as Weinstein (1998) points out, up until the late 1980s academic, professional and vocational education were held to be entirely discrete, with very different goals and designed for different groups of students.

National Vocational Qualifications

The NCVQ has prescribed a framework within which awarding bodies cast their regulations. This framework provides a two-dimensional classification for all qualifications by area of competence and level of performance. Providing health, social care and protective services is one specified area of competence. Other areas include tending animals, plants and the land; extracting and providing natural resources; and communicating.

NVQs are at five levels:

- *Level 1* relates to competence in performing a range of varied work activities, most of which are routine and predictable.
- *Level 2* relates to competence in a significant range of work activities, some of which are complex or non-routine, require some individual responsibility or autonomy and may require collaboration with others.
- *Level 3* relates to competence in a broad range of work activities, most of which are complex and non-routine. These activities are carried out in a range of contexts, involve considerable autonomy and responsibility for one's own work and that of others, and may involve allocation of resources.
- *Level 4* relates to competence which involves application of a significant

range of principles and complex techniques across a wide range of contexts which might be unpredictable. Work at this level involves considerable autonomy and significant responsibility for the work of others. Allocation of resources features strongly, as does personal accountability for analysis, diagnosis, planning, execution and evaluation.

In 1990 Level 5 competence was added to the existing four in preparation to include the professions.

● *Level 5* competence involves application of a significant range of fundamental principles and complex techniques across a wide range of occupational contexts; substantial personal autonomy and considerable responsibility for the work of others and for allocating resources; and personal accountability for analysis, diagnosis, planning, execution and evaluation.

The government's view set out in the white paper *Training for the 21st Century* (DES 1991) was that Level 5 should be introduced only when a comprehensive framework for Levels 1–4 was established, and that it would involve effective collaboration with professional bodies amongst others. In practice, distinguishing between competence at level 4 and 5 is difficult (Barr 1994).

The 1991 white paper (DES 1991) also equated NVQ levels with other vocational and academic qualifications:

● Level 1 – no equivalent vocational or academic qualifications
● Level 2 – Basic Craft Certificate, GCSE
● Level 3 – National Diploma, A levels
● Level 4 – Higher National Diploma, first degree
● Level 5 – no equivalent vocational award, postgraduate/professional

In the UK the government's national training and qualification targets were pursued through a complex structure of local Training and Enterprise Councils (TECs) and up to 160 lead industrial bodies. In 1993 these structures were rationalised and the lead industrial bodies were brought together under the Occupational Standards Councils. The Occupational Standards Council for Health and Social Care and the Care Sector Consortium encompassed six lead bodies within the health and social care field.

In spite of these changes progress towards the government's national training and vocational targets was slow. The government was concerned also about complaints by employers that a substantial proportion of the workforce lacked adequate core skills for employment (e.g. communication, numeracy, information technology). Part of the problem was perceived to be professional protectionism which impeded the access of students to awards and progression through them (Weinstein 1998). Most professions in the health and social care sector remained largely detached from the development of occupational standards and vocational qualifications apart from advising on the qualifications required by their support staff. An exception was psychology which was one of five pilot projects funded by NCVQ to develop higher level vocational qualifications.

Higher level NVQs and the response of the health professions

In 1994 the attention of the health and social care professions was focused sharply on National Standards developments and higher level vocational qualifications with a letter issued by the Secretary of State for Employment which raised the importance of fitting vocational awards coherently with academic and professional awards to ensure effective progression to full occupational competence at work. This letter was followed in 1995 by a consultation paper (DoE 1995) which explained the government's proposals to develop NVQs at levels 4 and 5. These initial proposals were heavily criticised by the professions and higher education interests which were concerned that methods of teaching and learning associated with S/NVQs at levels 1–3 were inappropriate at higher levels. Specifically they were concerned that such methods cannot address adequately the complexity of higher level roles and tasks, or provide students with sufficient depth and range of knowledge required for competent performance at higher levels. Further, there was concern that the NVQ approach to teaching and assessment cannot inculcate in students professional values or ethical perspectives, or the ability to initiate and manage change.

The government took account of the concerns of the professions and higher education in a position paper on higher vocational qualifications (DfEE 1996). Weinstein (1998) points out that this paper:

- Acknowledges the limitations of functional analysis as a method of describing higher level occupations
- Acknowledges that professionals require high level knowledge and that S/NVQ provides only a foundation for this knowledge base
- Differentiates clearly between simply remembering facts and understanding and applying knowledge in different settings
- Invites higher education institutions to play a major role in formulating and assessing higher level vocational qualifications
- Recognises the need for professionals to learn to problem solve, work through uncertainty and develop self awareness and skills for reflective practice
- Recognises that many practice professions (such as nursing) already assess practice competence in field placements and provide the knowledge to underpin competent practice through the academic curriculum
- Indicates that existing professional qualifications are unlikely to be changed radically or be replaced, although adjustment may be needed to bring them into line with the proposed national framework.

In summary, the relationship between vocational and academic and professional education of health and social care occupations is in a period of transition. Concerns remain among academics that NVQs are reductionist and anti-educational, and some professionals fear that occupational mapping and standards development will expose overlap between professional roles which will threaten professional roles and lower educational standards. However, the government seems to have made a genuine attempt to respond to these concerns and the 1996 position paper has been given a cautious welcome by the professions (H&CPEF 1996). The Dearing Report on higher education published in 1997 (DfEE 1997) emphasises the importance of education as a preparation for employment and the need for partnership between higher education, employers and the professions to ensure this. Thus the clear distinction that once existed between vocational, academic and professional education is a thing of the past.

Conclusion

At the beginning of this chapter we set out certain key issues which have dominated nurse education, in particular with regard to the nature of the preparation for professional practice as operationalised on both pre- and post-registration programmes.

The UKCC (1986) had argued that a theoretically-based approach to the initial preparation of nurses, in which students were educated to diploma level in institutions of higher education, would improve the quality and appropriateness of nurses' educational preparation and attract a broader range of new recruits (e.g. men and mature students). The initiative known as 'A New Preparation for Practice' (UKCC 1986) not only presented the profession's ambitions for a new preparation for nurses but also its vision of a so-called 'new' practitioner able to function effectively in an increasingly complex health care environment.

The pace of change incurred with the introduction of the DipHE programme has, however, been unprecedented and challenging, not least because subsequent educational reform has not only focused on the preparation of nurses for practice but has also impacted on the continuing professional development and education of nurses already entered onto the Register (UKCC 1994). Concerns had been expressed regarding the apparent lack of commitment in the UK to continuing professional education by both nurses and their employers for some time (e.g. Rogers 1987, Stanford 1989), a problem exacerbated by the speed of advancing technology rendering skills and knowledge obsolete. In addition, evidence was growing of the inequitable provision of continuing education opportunities to different groups of nurses such as part-time, junior and/or night nurses (Clarke & Rees 1989, Larcombe & Maggs 1991, Barriball & While 1996), confounding the profession's aspirations to nurture a commitment to life-long learning among all its members (ENB 1994).

Equally important is the increasing requirement for flexibility in the nursing workforce in order to meet the continually developing and changing needs of patients and clients, coupled with the organisational needs of an expanding health care service (Ham 1992). Post-registration nurse education with its focus on clinical skills acquisition is currently seen as a means of both remedying skills deficits and enhancing the scope of professional practice.

The future for nurse education remains uncertain. An increase in the number of three year nursing degree programmes looks set to continue, which poses questions regarding the future of the existing diploma programme. If, as appears likely, the latter acquires degree status in the not too distant future, the current broad entry gate will pose further problems. The development of National Vocational Qualifications to higher levels has blurred the clear distinction that once existed between academic, vocational and professional education. Furthermore, the inherent conflicts remain between the needs of service providers and the aspirations of nursing's professional body and nurse educators. The problems which have beset nurse education both at pre- and post-registration level appear therefore no nearer to resolution. In particular, the constant need to attract sufficient recruits to meet future service needs and to ensure sufficient numbers of appropriately skilled staff remains a consistent challenge, made more acute by the uneasy relationship between purchasers and providers of nurse education.

References

Akinsanya, J.A. (1990) Nursing links with higher education: a prescription for change in the 21st century. *Journal of Advanced Nursing*, 15, 744–54.

Alexander, M.F. (1983) *Learning to Nurse: Integrating Theory and Practice*. Churchill Livingstone, Edinburgh.

Atkins, S. & Williams, A. (1995) Registered nurses' experience of mentoring undergraduate nursing students. *Journal of Advanced Nursing*, 21, 1006–15.

Audit Commission (1986) *Making a Reality of community Care: A Report*. HMSO, London.

Barnett, D.E. (1981) Do nurses read. *Nursing Times*, 77(50), 2131–4.

Barr, H. (1994) NVQs and their implications for inter-professional collaboration. In *Going inter-professional* (ed. A. Leathard). Routledge, London.

Barriball, K.L. & While, A. (1996) Participation in continuing education in nursing: findings of an interview study. *Journal of Advanced Nursing*, 23, 999–1007.

Batstone, G. & Edwards, M. (1996) Professional roles in promoting evidence-based practice. *Management Review*, 2(3), 144–7.

Beckett, C. (1984) Student status in nursing: a discussion on the status of the student and how it affects training. *Journal of Advanced Nursing*, 9, 363–74.

Bell, P. (1983) *Initial nurse training: a historical perspective and an evaluation of the programme in three study hospitals*. Unpublished MSc Thesis. Cranfield Institute of Technology, Cranfield.

Bellone, C. (1996) On a role. *Nursing Times*, 92(51), 27–8.

Burnard, P. & Morrisson, P. (1991) Preferred learning and teaching strategies. (Brief research report.) *Nursing Times*, 87(9), 52.

Care Sector Consortium (1997) *National Occupational Standards for Professional Activity in Health Promotion and Care – Introductory Guide*. The Local Government Management Board, London.

Carlisle, C., Luker, K., Riley, E., Stilwell, J.A., Wilson, R. & Davies, C. (1996) *Skills*

Competency in Nursing Education: Adapting to Diploma Level Preparation in the Clinical Area. Conference paper presented at the British Educational Research Association Conference, University of Lancaster.

Carr-Hill, R., Dixon, P., Gibbs, I., Higgins, M., McCaughan, D. & Wright, K. (1992) *Skill Mix and the Effectiveness of Nursing Care*. Centre for Health Economics, University of York, York.

Carter, G.B. (1956) *A Study of the Course for Nurse Tutors Organised by the Royal College of Nursing (Scottish Branch) Leading to the Certificate Awarded by the University of Edinburgh*. Royal College of Nursing, London.

Centre for Health Economics (1995) *Fewer Doctors? More Nurses?* Centre for Health Economics, University of York, York.

Chapman, C. (1980) The learner as worker. *Medical Teacher*, **2**(5), 241–4.

Chiarella, M. (1990) Developing the credibility of continuing education. *Nurse Education Today*, 10, 70–73.

Clarke, J. & Rees, C. (1989) The midwife and continuing education. *Midwives Chronicle*, 102, 288–90.

Clifford, C. (1995) The role of nurse teachers: concerns, conflicts and challenges. *Nurse Education Today*, **15**(1), 11–16.

Collins, S.M. (1984) A broad overview of developments in nursing education and their implications for the delivery of nursing care. *International Journal of Nursing Studies*, **21**(3), 201–208.

Coopers & Lybrand (1995) *Nurse Practitioner Project*. Commissioned by the NHS Executive. Coopers & Lybrand, London.

Crotty, M. & Butterworth, T. (1992) The emerging role of the nurse teacher in Project 2000 programmes in England: a literature review. *Journal of Advanced Nursing*, 17, 1377–87.

David, A. (1994) Worth their salt. *Nursing Times*, **90**(51), 14.

Davidoff, F., Haynes, B., Sackett, D. & Smith R. (1995) Evidence based medicine. *British Medical Journal*, **6987**(310), 1085–6.

Dean, D. (1987) *Manpower Solutions*. Scutari Projects Ltd, London.

Deighan, M. & Hitch, S. (eds) (1995) *Clinical Effectiveness: From Guidelines to Cost-Effective Practice*. Earlybrave Publications, Brentwood.

Denner, S. (1995) Extending professional practice: benefits and pitfalls. *Nursing Times*, **91**(14), 27–9.

DES (Department of Education and Science) (1991) *Education and training for the 21st Century*, Vols 1 and 2. HMSO, London.

DfEE (Department of Education and Employment((1997) *Report of the National Committee of Inquiry into Higher Education* (chaired by Sir Ron Dearing). The Stationery Office, London.

DHSS (Department of Health and Social Security) (1972) *Report of the Committee on Nursing*. Cmnd 5115. (chairman Mr Briggs). HMSO, London.

DoE (Department of Employment) (1995) *A vision for higher level vocational qualifications*. HMSO, London.

DoH (Department of Health) (1989) *Working for Patients: Education and Training*. Working Paper 10. HMSO, London.

DoH (Department of Health) (1991) *Junior Doctors' Hours: The New Deal*. HMSO, London.

DoH (Department of Health) (1992) *Health of the Nation*. HMSO, London.

DoH (Department of Health) (1994) *Nursing, Midwifery and Health Visiting Education: A Statement of Strategic Intent*. HMSO, London.

Dowling, S., Barrett, S. & West, R. (1995) With nurse practitioners, who needs house officers? *British Medical Journals*, 311, 309–13.

Dunn, L. (1997) A literature review of advanced clinical nursing practice in the United States of America. *Journal of Advanced Nursing*, 25, 814–19.

Edwards, R., Sieminski, S. & Zeldin, D. (eds) (1993) *Adult Learners, Education and Training*, Routledge, London.

Elkan, R. (1995) Project 2000: a review of the published research. *Journal of Advanced Nursing*, 22, 386–92.

Elkan, R., Hillman, R. & Robinson, J. (1993) *The implementation of Project 2000 in a district health authority: the effect on the nursing service.* Second Interim Report. Dept of Nursing and Midwifery Studies, University of Nottingham, Nottingham.

Elkan, R., Hillman, R. & Robinson, J. (1995) How does P2000 affect staffing levels. *Nursing Times*, **91**(3), 11–12.

Elkan, R. & Robinson, J. (1993) Project 2000: the gap between theory and practice. *Nurse Education Today*, 13, 295–8.

ENB (1989) *Project 2000 – A New Preparation for Practice: Guidelines and Criteria for Course Development.* English National Board for Nursing, Midwifery and Health Visiting, London.

ENB (1991) *Circular: Evaluation of three-year undergraduate nursing and midwifery programmes.* English National Board for Nursing, Midwifery and Health Visiting, London.

ENB (1994) *Creating Lifelong Learners: Partnerships for Care.* English National Board for Nursing, Midwifery and Health Visiting, London.

Eraut, M. (1994) *Developing professional knowledge and competence.* Falmer Press, London.

Fish, D., Twinn, S. & Purr, B. (1991) *Promoting reflection: improving the supervision of practice in health visiting and initial teacher training: how to enable students to learn through professional practice.* Report No. 2. West London Institute of Higher Education, London.

Fitzpatrick, J., While, A. & Roberts, J. (1993) The relationship between nursing and higher education. *Journal of Advanced Nursing*, 18, 1488–97.

French, P. (1989) *An assessment of the pre-registration preparation of nurses as an educational experience.* Unpublished PhD thesis. University of Durham, Durham.

Fretwell, J.E. (1980) An inquiry into the ward learning environment. *Nursing Times*, 76(16), 69–73.

Fretwell, J.E. (1983) Creating a ward learning environment: the sister's role part 1. *Nursing Times*, **79**(33), 37–9.

Fretwell, J.E. (1985) *Freedom to Change.* Royal College of Nursing, London.

Gillan, J. (1995) Editorial. *Nursing Times*, **91**(30), 24.

GNC (1969) *Guide to the Syllabus of Examination of the General Register.* General Nursing Council, London.

Greenhalgh Report (1994) *The Interface between Junior Doctors and Nurses: A Research Study for the Department of Health.* Greenhalgh and Co, London.

Greenwood, J. (1993) The apparent desensitization of student nurses during their professional socialisation: a cognitive perspective. *Journal of Advanced Nursing*, 18(9), 1471–9.

Ham, C. (1992) *Health Policy in Britain: the Politics and Organisation of the National Health Service*, (3rd edn.) Macmillan, Basingstoke.

Hamill, C. (1995) The phenomenon of stress as perceived by Project 2000 student nurses: a case study. *Journal of Advanced Nursing*, **21**(3), 528–36.

Hamilton, H. (1993) Care improves while costs reduce: the clinical nurse specialist in total parental nutrition. *Professional Nurse*, **8**(9), 592–4, 596.

Hammond, C., Chase, J. & Hogbin, B. (1995) A unique service? *Nursing Times*, **9**(30), 28–9.

Health and Care Professionals Education Forum (H & CPEF) (1996) Personal communication. Cited in Weinstein 1998.

Higgins, M. (1997) Developing and supporting expansion of the nurse's role. *Nursing Standard*, **11**(24), 41–4.

Hoover, J. & van Ooijen, E. (1995) Back to basics? *Nursing Times*, **91**(33), 42–43.

Houltram, B. (1996) Entry age, entry mode and academic performance on a Project 2000 common foundation programme. *Journal of Advanced Nursing*, 23, 1089–97.

Humphreys, J. (1995) The marketing gap in health care education. *Nurse Education Today*, 15, 202–209.

Humphreys, J. (1966a) Education commissioning by consortia: some theoretical and practical issues relating to qualitative aspects of British nurse education. *Journal of Advanced Nursing*, **24**(16), 1288–99.

Humphreys, J. (1996b) British National Health Service chief executives on nurse education: corporate instrumentalism and doubts on quasi-market structure. *Journal of Advanced Nursing*, **23**(1), 160–70.

Jacka, K. & Lewin, D. (1987) *The clinical learning of student nurses*. Report No 6. Nursing research Unit, King's College, University of London, London.

Jinks, A.M. (1994) Conceptualization of different levels of educational attainment: what are the characteristics of nurses and midwives who have undertaken diploma and degree educational programmes? *Journal of Nursing Management*, 2, 279–85.

Jones, E.G. (1996) *Interpretation of academic level three for nursing practice*. Unpublished MSc thesis. University of Cambridge, Cambridge.

Jones, W. (1981) Self-directed learning and student centred goals in nurse education *Journal of Advanced Nursing*, 16, 59–69.

Jordan, S. (1993) Nurse practitioners. Learning from the USA experience: a review of the literature. *Health and Social Care*, 2, 173–85.

Jowett, S. (1995) *A longitudinal interview study with Project 2000 students: their views and experiences during and after the course*. Unpublished PhD thesis. University of London, London.

Jowett, S., Walton, I. & Payne, S. (1992a) *The introduction of Project 2000: early perspectives from the students*. Interim Paper No. 5. National Foundation for Education Research in England and Wales, Slough.

Jowett, S., Walton, I. & Payne, S. (1992b) *The introduction of Project 2000: early perspectives from higher education*. Interim Paper No. 4. National Foundation for Educational Research in England and Wales, Slough.

Jowett, S., Walton, I. & Payne, S. (1994) *Challenges and Change in Nurse Education: A Study of the Implementation of Project 2000*. National Foundation for Educational Research in England and Wales, Slough.

Keep, E. (1993) Missing, presumed skills training policy in the United Kingdom. In: *Adult Learners, Education and Training*, (eds R. Edwards, S. Sieminski & D. Zeldin). Routledge, London.

Kemp, I. & Seagraves, L. (1995) Transferable skills – can higher education deliver? *Studies in Higher Education*, **20**(3), 315–28.

Kenrick, M.A. (1993) The problem of motivating teaching staff in a complex amalgamation. *Journal of Advanced Nursing*, 18, 1498–504.

Knowles, M. (1990) *The Adult Learner: A Neglected Species*, (4th edn). Gulf Publishing Company, Houston.

Lancet Commission on Nursing. (1932) Final Report. *Lancet*, I, 415.

Land, L., Mhaolrunaigh, S. & Castledine, G. (1996) Extent and effectiveness of the Scope of Professional Practice. *Nursing Times*, **92**(35), 32–5.

Larcombe, K. & Maggs, C. (1991) *Processes for Identifying the Continuing Education Needs of Nurses: An Evaluation*. ENB, London.

Lathlean, J. (1989) *Policy Making in Nurse Education*. Ashdale Press, Oxford.

Lathlean, J. & Farnish, S. (1984) *Ward Sister Training Project*. Chelsea College, Nursing Education Research Unit, London.

Lawson, P. & Emmerson, P. (1995) Nurse practitioners: agents of change. *Health Visitor*, **68**(6), 244–5.

Le Grand, J. & Bartlett, W. (eds) (1992) *Quasi-Markets and Social Policy*. Macmillan, London.

Logan, W. (1987) Is education for a nursing elite? Some highlights in nursing education in Europe and North America. *Nurse Education Today*, 7, 5–9.

Luker, K., Carlisle, C. & Kirk, S. (1995) *The Evolving Role of the Nurse Teacher in the Light of Educational Reforms*. ENB, London.

Mackereth, P. (1989) Investigation of the developmental influences on nurses' motivation for their continuing education. *Journal of Advanced Nursing*, 14, 776–87.

Macleod-Clark, J., Maben, J. & Jones, K. (1996) *Project 2000: Perceptions of the Philosophy and Practice of Nursing*. ENB, London.

Maguire, M. (1994) *The job of educating teachers*. Unpublished PhD Thesis. University of London.

Manpower Services Commission & Department for Education and Science (1986) *Review of Vocational Qualifications in England and Wales*. HMSO, London.

Marsh, G.N. & Dawes, M.L. (1995) Establishing a minor illness nurse in a busy general practice. *British Medical Journal*, 310, 778–80.

McMahon, F. & Carter, E. (1990) The great training robbery. Falmer Press, London.

Melia, K.M. (1987) *Learning and Working: the Occupational Socialisation of Nurses*. Tavistock Publications, London.

Miles, R., Skeath, A. & Tossel, D. (1988) *Management in Nurse Education*. Costello, Tunbridge Wells.

Miller, C., Jones, M. & Tomlinson, A. (1994) *The current teaching provision for individual learning styles of students on pre-registration diploma programmes in adult nursing*. Research Highlights No. 9. ENB, London.

Mitchell, L. & Cuthbert, T. (1989) Insufficient evidence? *The final report of the competency testing project*. SCOTVEC, Glasgow.

MoH (Ministry of Health) (1947) *Report of the Working Party on the Recruitment and Training of Nurses* (Chairman Sir R. Wood). HMSO, London.

Moores, B. & Moult, A. (1979) Patterns of nurse activity. *Journal of Advanced Nursing*, 4, 137–49.

Myco, F. (1980) Nursing research information: are nurse educators and practitioners seeking it out? *Journal of Advanced Nursing*, 5, 637–46.

Nemes, J. (1994) Nurse practitioners in acute care units. *Nursing Standard*, **9**(8), 37–40.

NHS (NHS Executive) (1996) *Education and Training Planning Guidance*. Department of Health, Leeds.

NHS (National Health Service) (1990) *NHS and Community Care Act*. HMSO, London.

O'Brien, D. & Heyman, B. (1989) Changes in nurse education and the facilitation of nursing research: an exploratory study. *Nurse Education Today*, 9, 392–6.

Ogier, M.E. (1982) *An Ideal Ward Sister: a Study of the Leadership Style and Verbal*

Interactions of Ward Sisters and Nurse Learners in General Hospitals. Royal College of Nursing, London.

OPCS (Office of Population, Censuses and Surveys) (1987) *Population Projections No 16*. HMSO, London.

OPCS (Office of Population, Censuses and Surveys) (1989) *Social Trends, No 19*. HMSO, London.

OPCS (Office of Population Census and Surveys) (1991) *Qualified Nurses, Midwives and Health Visitors*. HMSO, London.

OPCS (Office of Population, Censuses and Surveys) (1994) *Social Trends, No 24*. HMSO, London.

Orton, H.D. (1981) *Ward Learning Climate: a Study of the Role of the Ward Sister in Relation to Student Nurse Learning on the Ward*. Royal College of Nursing, London.

Payne, S., Jowett, S. & Walton, I. (1991) *Nurse teachers in Project 2000: the experience of planning and initial implementation*. Interim Paper No 3. National Foundation for Educational Research in England and Wales, Slough.

Pearson, K., Kelly, A., Connolly, M., Daly, M. & O'Gorman, F. (1995) Nurse practitioners. *Health Visitor*, **68**(4), 157–60.

Phillips, T., Shostack, J., Bedford, H. & Robinson, J. (1993) *Assessment of Competencies in Nursing and Midwifery Education and Training (the Ace Project)*. Research Highlights. ENB, London.

Ramprogus, V. (1995) *The Destruction of Nursing: Developments in Nursing and Health Care*. Avebury, Aldershott.

RCN (1942) *Nursing Reconstruction Committee* (Chairman, Lord Horder). Royal College of Nursing, London.

RCN/NCN (1964) *A Reform of Nursing Education*. First report of a special committee on nurse education (Chairman Sir H. Platt). Royal College of Nursing and National Council for Nurses of the United Kingdom, London.

RCN/NCN (1985) *The Education of Nursing: a new dispensation*. Report of the Commission of Nurse Education. (Chairman: Mr Harry Judge). Royal College of Nursing and National Council for Nurses of the United Kingdom, London.

Rees, M. & Kinnersley, P. (1996) Nurse-led management of minor illness in a GP surgery. *Nursing Times*, **92**(6), 32–3.

Reid, N.G. (1985) *Ward in Chancery?* Royal College of Nursing, London.

Reid, N., Todd, C. & Robinson, G. (1991) Educational activities on wards under 12 hour shifts. *International Journal of Nursing Studies*, **28**(1), 47–54.

Robinson, J. (1991a) Project 2000: evaluating the courses. *Nursing Times*, **87**(21), 29–30.

Robinson, J. (1991b) *The First Year – Experience of a Project 2000 Demonstration District*. Suffolk and Great Yarmouth College of Nursing and Midwifery, Ipswich.

Robinson, J. (1992) Mixed feelings. *Nursing Times*, **88**(40), 28–30.

Rogers, J. (1987) Limited opportunities. *Nursing Times*, **83**(36), 31–2.

Roques, A. (1996) Contract to learn. *Nursing Times*, **92**(35), 52–3.

Rosenholtz, S.J. (1989) *Schools, Social Organisation and the Building of a Technical Culture*. Longman, New York.

Schön, D. (1983) *The Reflective Practitioner: How Professionals Think*. Temple Smith, London.

Sloan, J.P. & Slevin, O.D. (1991) *Teaching and Supervision of Student Nurses During Practice Placements*. National Board for Nursing, Midwifery and Health Visiting for N. Ireland.

Smith, A. & Jacobsen, B. (1988) *The Nation's Health: a Strategy for the 1990s*. King's Fund, London.

Stanford, J. (1989) Continuing education. *Journal of District Nursing*, 7 (April), 8–10, 12.

Stanwick, S. (1994) The market for education: supply and demand. In: *Health Care Education: The Challenge of the Market*, (eds J. Humphreys & F.M. Quinn), pp. 102–17. Chapman & Hall, London.

Statutory Instrument No. 1456 (1989) *The Nurses, Midwives and Health Visitors (Registered Fever Nurses Amendment Rules and Training Amendment Rules) Approval Order*. HMSO, London.

Studdy, S. & Hunt, C. (1980) A computerised survey of learning needs. *Nursing Times*, **76**(25), 1084–7.

Sutton, F. & Smith, C. (1995) Advanced nursing practice: new ideas and new perspectives. *Journal of Advanced Nursing*, 21, 1037–43.

Telford, W. (1979) Determining nursing establishments. *Health Service Manpower Review*, **5**(4), 11–17.

Thomason, G. (1988) *A Textbook of Human Resource Management*. Institute of Personnel Management, London.

Touche Ross Management Consultants (1995) *Evaluation of Nurse Practitioner Pilot Projects*. NHS Executive/RHA, South Thames, London.

Trnobranski, P.H. (1994) Nurse practitioner: redefining the role of the community nurse? *Journal of Advanced Nursing*, 19, 134–9.

UKCC (1980) *Annual Report*. United Kingdom Central Council for Nursing, Midwifery and Health Visiting, London.

UKCC (1982) *The development of nurse education*. Working Group 3, Consultation Paper 1, Education and Training. United Kingdom Central Council for Nursing, Midwifery and Health Visiting, London.

UKCC (1985) *Project 2000: student status revisited*. Project Paper 2. United Kingdom Central Council for Nursing, Midwifery and Health Visiting, London.

UKCC (1986) *Project 2000: a new preparation for practice*. United Kingdom Central Council for Nursing, Midwifery and Health Visiting, London.

UKCC (1987) *P2000: The Final Proposals*. United Kingdom Central Council for Nursing, Midwifery and Health Visiting, London.

UKCC (1988) *UKCC's Proposed Rules for the Standard, Kind and Content of Future Pre-Registration Nursing Education*. United Kingdom Central Council for Nursing, Midwifery and Health Visiting, London.

UKCC (1992a) *The Scope of Professional Practice*. United Kingdom Central Council for Nursing, Midwifery and Health Visiting, London.

UKCC (1992b) *Code of Professional Conduct*, (3rd edn). United Kingdom Central Council for Nursing, Midwifery and Health Visiting, London.

UKCC (1992c) *Exercising Accountability*. United Kingdom Central Council for Nursing, Midwifery and Health Visiting, London.

UKCC (1994) *The Future of Professional Practice – the Council's Standards for Education and Practice Following Registration*. United Kingdom Central Council for Nursing, Midwifery and Health Visiting, London.

UKCC (1998) *A higher level of practice*. Consultation document. United Kingdom Central Council for Nursing, Midwifery and Health Visiting, London.

Vaughan, B. (1989) Autonomy and accountability. *Nursing Times*, **85**(3), 54–5.

Wade, B. & Moyer, A. (1989) An evaluation of clinical nurse specialists: implications for education and organisation of care. *Senior Nurse*, **9**(9), 11–16.

Waters, J. (1996) Dorrell denies crisis in nurse recruitment. *Nursing Times*, **92**(30) 10.

Watson, P., Hendey, N. & Dingwell, R. (1994) *Role extension/expansion with particular reference to the nurse practitioner: A review of the literature*. University of Nottingham, Nottingham.

Weight, T. (1996) Educational purchasing consortia. *Health Service Manager*, 10, 3–4.

Weinstein, J. (1998) The use of National Occupational Standards in professional education. *Journal of Interprofessional Care*, **12**(2), 169–79.

West Midlands RHA (1995) *Advanced Nurse Practitioner Programmes*. RHA and Birmingham University, West Midlands.

While, A.E., Roberts, J.D. & Fitzpatrick, J.M. (1995) *A Comparative Study of Outcomes of Pre-Registration Nurse Education Programmes*. ENB, London.

White, E., Riley, E., Davies, S. & Twinn, S. (1994) *A Detailed Study of the Relationship between Teaching, Support, Supervision and Role Modelling in Clinical Areas, Within the Context of Project 2000 Courses*. ENB, London.

Wilson-Barnett, J. (1995) Specialism in nursing: effectiveness and maximisation of benefit. *Journal of Advanced Nursing*, 21, 1–2.

Wilson-Barnett, J. & Beech, S. (1994) Evaluating the clinical nurse specialist: a review. *International Journal of Nursing Studies*, **31**(6), 561–71.

Witz, A. (1994) The challenge of nursing. In: *Challenging Medicine*, (eds J. Gabe, D. Kelleher & D. Williams), pp. 23–45. Routledge, London.

Wright, S. (1995) The role of the nurse: extended or expanded? *Nursing Standard*, **9**(33), 25–29.

Section 4
Nursing: The Reality

Commentary: Present Realities and Future Directions

This book opened by setting the debates and reasons for whether nursing should continue to aspire to a future as a 'profession', or if it would better serve the needs of the public and contribute to human well-being by casting itself in the mould of managerialism. The two chapters in the first section of the book presented the case for the professionalists, while the four chapters in the second section were more favourably disposed towards a managerial option. However, neither approach seems able to offer the complete answer, perhaps because the old-fashioned legacies of both traditions hamper forward thinking, or because of fears and conflicts on either side.

This dilemma is confronted in this final section, which returns to the idea raised in the introduction, of two different discourses existing side by side but never quite managing to engage in constructive dialogue. The two chapters come from different perspectives, to explore whether it is possible to draw together positive, forward looking ideas from both approaches, and merge them into a new view of nursing as an occupation.

In Chapter 8, Bergen revisits the arguments she raised earlier in the book. Professionals do not practise in the abstract but in real settings, engaging with real people. Rather than asserting simply that caring is the core of nursing practice, she argues that a convincing analysis must take account of the historical, social, organisational and political contexts within which it is practised. In essence, the ethical and social basis from which the occupation derives the right to practise is what matters, not whether it is regarded as a profession or not. Thus, Bergen looks at the institutions that employ nurses and sets them in the context of the wider society that establishes those organisations. The way they are set up says something about the societies, and nurses would do well to heed the hidden messages about the position they are deemed to hold.

The second chapter in this concluding section (Chapter 9) looks outwards from nursing to the wider setting. Edwards and Hale shift the debate to a consideration of professions and health policy. The position of nursing in relation to a multiprofessional workforce is considered, as is the need for a much clearer research base to underpin nursing work. Paradoxically, both these aspects require a clear professional identity if the essential needs of the patients being served are not to be submerged in the wider agenda of the organisation. Thus, organisations need to support and respect the professional knowledge of nursing; nursing in turn must contribute more positively to developing that base.

These two chapters each demonstrate the importance of heeding the alternative viewpoint, and draw the text to a close. The book has high-lighted four key areas on which nursing may wish to concentrate as it maps a course for itself, which combine the benefits of both a professional and managerial outlook:

(1) The ethical basis and key reason for employing nurses both stem from the nature of the service that can be delivered. Any claim for occupational advancement, therefore, should only be made from the perspective of the recipient of the services, not from that of the nurses.

(2) This leads on to the need for nurses to develop their own capacity and that of co-workers, colleagues, team members and clients. There is no exclusive knowledge base, but sharing and working towards a highly developed and differentiated multidisciplinary knowledge offers the highest potential.

(3) Nursing should extend its remit from a focus on the therapeutic input to a single recipient of care, to explore its potential across the wider field of health care. This would mean accepting and expecting to take responsibility for assuring overall quality through multiple means, facilitating and delegating as well as delivering hands-on care.

(4) Finally, the importance of developing the knowledge base of how high quality care is assured and what is meant by 'successful nursing' across fields cannot be emphasised enough. There is a role for nursing in developing its own knowledge base and in contributing to a multidisciplinary awareness of the relevance and use of evidence-based practice.

All the contributors to this book are either academic staff or post-graduate students in the Florence Nightingale Division of Nursing and Midwifery at King's College London. Most are members of the Health Care Education and Professional Development Research Group, at a meeting of which the idea for the book was born. We are grateful to all our colleagues for taking time out of their busy lives to contribute to this project, and look forward to continuing the debate as we strive towards excellence in nursing practice, education and research.

8 Nursing as Caring Revisited

Ann Bergen

Nursing, like teaching (though not necessarily the two combined), is one of those occupations that seldom calls for clarification when given as a response to the person-defining question, 'What do you do?'. It would seem that everyone, from little girls with their career aspirations mapped out, to politicians legislating for health care, intuitively 'know' what nursing is.

Sadly, such intuitive 'knowledge' is often found wanting. There is evidence that, even today, public and media images of nurses and nursing fail to reflect reality. A recent review of references to nursing in *The Higher* (latterly *The Times Higher Educational Supplement*) found them to be 'disappointingly stereotypical, framed within a medical model, with female nurses, frilly hats and hospital equipment illustrating articles which focus on change' (Miers 1996, p. 20). More recently still, a British Health Minister Gerald Malone attracted censure from nursing unions for his claim that nursing has an image as it is portrayed in the 'Carry On' films of yesteryear – 'all mops and bedpans' (*Nursing Standard* 1996).

But images of nursing are probably easier to demolish than to construct. In seeking 'the reality' of nursing, a useful starting point is perhaps to be found in the ideals underpinning its practice, as identified in Chapter 3. Yet, on their own, there is a danger that these ideals could lead to the popular misconceptions highlighted above. The title of this book, together with the previous chapters, suggest that the actual practice of nursing is highly complex and much influenced by its context, particularly the managerial and organisational contexts, but also the political, social and historical forces at work behind these. This chapter aims to review some of these contextual variables with respect to their influences on nursing's caring ideals, in order to further clarify the reality of nursing.

The role of context

While the influence of context on any ideology in its outworking is indisputable, the extent to which this may actually define reality is more open to argument, as are the ways in which contextual influences are manifest. For instance, Fealy (1995) sees the bases of caring as being in the carer's perception of the self-perceived needs of individuals in a given situation and at a given time. Caring, to this writer, is about individual moral decisions and acts which also have external influences. But Fealy also acknowledges that this stance cuts across the Kantian ethic of the 'categorical imperative' – the idea that an action is deemed good (or not) based on universal principle, rather than on its outcome or particular circumstances. This argument is supported by other theorists who view caring from a moral viewpoint. Lea & Watson (1996) point out that nurse theorists Watson and Leininger do not believe that caring as nursing practice should change from one patient to another.

Both sides of this debate have credence. On the one hand, a claim to universality of principle may bolster claims to uniqueness of a discipline or profession – something particularly attractive, perhaps, to an occupation like nursing at a time it is seeking to establish its particular contribution to health care. On the other hand, such claims may be difficult to uphold in a practice-based discipline and a number of commentators, through either empirical studies or reviews of the literature, have noted the potential discrepancy between ideals and reality to which this may give rise.

Benner & Wrubel (1989), for instance, in asserting that caring is not context free, point out that theory must be informed by real world experiences – a stance which itself informs, and is informed by, their inductive research paradigm. Similarly, Smith (1992), in her study of emotional labour in nursing, prefaced her book with an account of the motivation to undertake an in-depth study of the subjective experiences of student nurses; this comprised a questioning of whether she was teaching to strive for ideals that, although prompted by popular nursing ideology, were inappropriate to everyday realities. Clifford (1995) makes a similar point in a review of caring, pointing out the limitations of conceptual analyses without reference to the real world of practice:

'whilst many of the texts in caring in nursing explore the process of nursing, they tend to do so in isolation from the world in which nurses work and the factors that promote nurses to work in that environment.'

(Clifford, 1995, p. 39)

Such an argument is given weight through a consideration of some of the variables which impact on the operationalisation of ideals. Benner & Wrubel (1989) talk about power relations which create particular conditions, while Fealy (1995) mentions social, cultural and historical criteria. Perry (1993) goes so far as to say that the reality of nursing and caring is actually the product of history and social practices, rather than anything to do with logic, though this again begs the question of the extent to which pragmatics can legitimately override ideals in terms of defining the essence of a practice discipline. Some of these variables will be explored in greater depth presently.

One possible way of safeguarding against extremist positions on either side of this debate is suggested by Warelow (1996). While seeing caring as context dependent and related to the 'prevailing unique circumstances' (p.655), the author also suggests reality is found in the moral dimension of the concept. However, unlike Kant, Warelow adopts a teleological rather than a deontological position, indicating that an action is judged as caring (or not) by its consequences, in terms of meeting the presenting needs of any given patient, client, family or group. This is consonant with the assertion of Cox (1993) that values should determine practice in nursing, insofar as specific interventions should be based on whether they are in the interests of patients/clients. It also accommodates Brykczynska's (1993) suggestion that nurses may at times have espoused certain values that, at best, have outlived their usefulness; values, in other words, are useful as guidelines to practice, but their relevance is determined by anticipated ends, not as means in themselves. This point can be illustrated by looking at nursing's historical context.

The historical context

It is probably true to say that, over time, nursing has been governed by differing emphases, if not actual principles. Preceding chapters, for instance, have noted a British nursing focus on the instrumental aspects of its practice some 30 to 40 years ago (Bradshaw 1995) and an influence of the counselling ideology which popularised humanistic ideals in the 1960s (Campbell 1984). Both manifestations may have been appropriate in their time and place and neither necessarily have any *a priori* claim to represent the reality of nursing.

Jolley (1993) further illustrates and develops this point convincingly in a consideration of historical influences on nursing, traced back to Florence Nightingale. Nightingale, claims Jolley, was able to transform and elevate the image of the nurse through her image as a national heroine during a period when heroic-type activities appealed to the dominant value system. While this represented, perhaps, only one side of the coin – the 'strong, ruthless, manipulative, aggressive and neurotic personality' was largely ignored along with other less desirable traits – it was appropriate to the time, as was the concept of the ordinary nurse as a member of the servant class, 'subordinate, servile, humble, self-sacrificing and not too learned' (p.11). Thus emerged the inferior status of nursing in the power relationship with the medical profession – a relationship which mirrored the female/male, probationer/lady pupil and nurse/superintendent relationship and the very unequal social class divisions of contemporary Victorian society.

But, continues Jolley (1993), 'what gave rise to problems in the decades that followed was the determined maintenance of, and clinging to, a tradition and image, parts of which, as the 19th century progressed, were to become increasingly non-viable' (p.15). By the early 20th century the medical professional dominance and sexual role stereotypes were still in existence and, indeed, could be said to be so today judging by the media portrayals discussed at the start of this chapter.

There is, of course, the danger of adopting the opposite position and, as it were, throwing the baby out with the bathwater. So how should contemporary nurses react in setting an appropriate agenda for nursing which maintains a balance between its ideals and its historical legacy?

Brykczynska (1993) quotes Thoreau's observation that one generation tends to abandon the enterprises of another like stranded vessels, and suggests, as a possible way forward, that perhaps it would be more profitable if we 'simply re-examined the values of our past and saw what was good and wholesome, what is, therefore, worth retaining, and what will need to be modified or abandoned' (p.155). Thoughtful counsel undoubtedly, but needing to be operationalised within the related social and cultural context.

Social and cultural context

Sociologists advise us that social and cultural contexts have significant influence over individuals', and even a profession's, behaviour. Jolley (1993) comments that 'institutions and professions reflect, within their own structures, the society in which they have their own being, including pre-vailing norms, attitudes, beliefs and values' (p. 1). This, of course, begs the question of whether nurses, either individually or collectively, have the ability and will to manipulate these influences, as they may perhaps discount historical tradition, in forging a reality for nursing.

Much of the literature would suggest not. In particular, it suggests nurses and nursing might find it difficult to influence positive images of nursing in a society where the values it embodies are not recognised. Benner & Wrubel (1989) comment that their book was written in the context of the highly technical and individualistic culture of the US, during a time of acute nursing shortage. The way that caring had become suspect in a climate where self-care was the ideal made for a general societal devaluation of nursing.

The influence of social factors can also be detected in research in the UK. Smith (1992), in her study of emotional labour in nursing, described a 'pecking order' of clinical experience, which reflects the societal view of placing high value on 'high tech' medicine, and the marginalisation of the caretaking activities which characterise caring for the elderly and chronically ill. Further, both Pendleton (1993) and Warelow (1996) highlight the seminal work of Melia (1987) which demonstrated how student nurses were socialised into the prevailing value system during training; 'fitting in' often took precedence over patient care. Warelow (1996) comments that nursing practice is thus likely to be determined by the group rather than any ideals of education, and that if caring is context dependent, then to 'fit in' means going with the consensus rather than upholding individual ethical ideals. Not that this negates the ethical dimension of caring in itself (as discussed in Chapter 3) if, as Warelow (1996) seems to imply, there exists a corporate professional value system. But, he states:

> 'One of the central dilemmas in the nursing profession is the moral question of being ordered or expected to care in a society that refuses to value caring.'

> (Warelow, 1996, p. 659)

It is rather the adoption of one universalised theoretical ethical position which Warelow sees as being unrealistic and unwise.

Social influences may also serve as a 'hidden agenda' in nursing, according to Perry's (1993) reading of the issue. She describes the 'hidden rules' of a social structure which supports the separation of care and cure and maintains nursing in its 'handmaiden mentality'. It also puts nursing in the somewhat paradoxical role of being marginal to medical and scientific endeavour, yet central to medical health practices (especially when medical professionals are absent and nurses function independently). Further, argues Perry (1993), these 'hidden agendas' reveal that social institutions have different ways of valuing people apart from openly stated rules and 'the assumptions which inform this differential evaluation of occupational groups are located in a class-bound society' (p. 68). These factors maintain nursing as an 'under-profession' (Perry's preferred term to semi-profession), overshadowed by medical and governmental definitions of its interests.

It could be argued, of course, that this view overplays the role of the impersonal, general forces at the expense of the individuals who constitute the nursing profession. As Brykczynska (1993) points out, in a pluralistic society not everyone places the same values on potential norms, benefits and prohibitions and, in reality, there may be few shared values in nursing, especially at the trans-cultural and international levels. Perry (1993) herself comments that nurses have to make these work prescriptions, meted out by the hidden social structure, a reality. Moreover, she states, nurses serve, not an abstract entity called a health organisation, but the interests of real people in a real setting. Lawler (1991) also sees limitations in the macro-level sociological analysis approach to describing the reality of nursing. The basis of her 'somological' account of nursing – knowledge derived from practical, professional experience – lay in tapping the everyday work of individual nurses, dealing with people through their own accounts of practice which were 'interpretative, contextual and integrative of subject and object' (p.5). Her major concepts and parameters of nursing were built on these accounts.

If nursing, then, must be defined in terms of both its overall social construction and the different individuals who constitute its varying practices, then intermediate structures should, perhaps, also inform the debate. Thus, different specialisms within the profession, though operating in the same society, can, like individuals, carve out their own realities appropriate to them. The specialist paediatric oncology nurses described by Bignold *et al.* (1995) identified 'befriending' as a concept useful to their particular practice. However, the researchers of their role caution that, while there may be analogies made with other spheres of nursing practice, it will not serve as a universal ideal.

As with its relationship with historical tradition, then, nursing in practice must necessarily accommodate the realities of the social context in its outworkings. Nurses, as Clifford (1995) says, must acknowledge that they are paid for what they do and subject to the controls imposed by the health care system. Nurses are fulfilling a social role, designed to meet the identified needs of society, and this is inevitably more circumscribed than the general idealistic notion of caring in its altruistic guise. The construct of 'formalized caring' (Clifford 1995), discussed previously, is therefore probably a useful notion for nurses to adopt, since, while it acknowledges a diversity in practice, it also recognises there are boundaries to the nursing contribution to caring in society. The balance for practitioners of nursing, in steering a path which embraces ideals and social demands, is also, however, mediated by the more immediate organisational context.

Organisational context

Although the literature suggests there is no consensus regarding the extent and nature of the effects of organisational structure on nursing practice, it does overwhelmingly indicate it to be a force to be considered. Chapters 4 to 6 of this book have examined some of the organisational and managerial factors, both internal and external to nursing, which have influenced its development, while Chapter 7 has looked at how nurse education has risen to the challenge of preparing practitioners to work in the resulting context. This section will focus more specifically on how these factors have been conducive or detrimental to nurses realising the caring ideal outlined in Chapter 3.

Caring, as has been seen, is often depicted as a relationship, and Wade (1995), in looking at nursing care as a relationship based on partnership between client and nurse, believes that the organisational environment, in terms of the hospital or health centre, can often negatively influence this ideal. Organisational and resource constraints, giving rise to such features as shorter hospital stays, the increase in day surgery, the reduction in long stay care facilities and high degrees of patient movement, have led, in her view, to an environment which is intimidating to service users and may lead to conformity, rather than individuality, in care practices.

Webb (1996) picks up the issue of resource constraints which may characterise certain organisational settings and thereby affect care, or, more particularly, the balance between care and cure, the affective and instrumental emphases of practice. Thus 'uncaring' – nursing which fails to reflect the ethical values of the caring concept – may be the result of insufficient resources to support good practice. However, the care/cure balance may also be due to the implementation of what is thought to be an appropriate response to nursing within a given organisational setting; Webb (1996) cites as an example here the difference found in studies between acute and long term wards for the elderly where 'cure' is often the yardstick applied to the former, but is not so appropriate to the latter.

Perry (1993) offers a similar, but more detailed, analysis of why current health care organisations are generally inimical to the promotion of individualised, holistically focused nurse–patient caring relationships. Such personalised caring, she notes, is expensive, political and 'invisible' in health institutions, forcing nurses to rely on more obvious instrumental demonstrations and measurements of caring, rather than their own definitions. Much caring expertise is, therefore, not recognised by the organisation or its value systems, and practitioners must resort to inconsistencies and double standards, and cope with the resulting conflict. The real role relationship for nurses, according to Perry's analysis, is not to be found between nurse and patient, but between nursing care and health administration. And in this relationship nurses have a relatively low status, such that the occupational role of caring is marginalised compared to technical and managerial expertise.

Interestingly, Perry (1993) also feels that the pervading management ethos takes precedence for nurses who become managers themselves, over the caring face of the profession:

'Nurses who become managers are managers first and foremost. Their definition of nursing problems and solutions arises out of organisational need rather than a preoccupation with nursing interventions and patients' rights to health.'

(Perry, 1993, p. 71)

She concludes that, even the advent of the 'new managerialism' in nursing does not necessarily mean that nurses have more say and responsibility in the way they carry out caring.

This inherent conflict between the nature of institutional structures and caring principles is also noted by Brykczynska (1993). In her view an institutional value system reflects the aggregated values of many different individuals solidified around a significant investment of time and energy. As such, this value system may conflict with individuals whose required behaviour is difficult to elicit, thus causing institutional performance to suffer. Once again, it appears the caring ideals of nursing may be compromised, and nurses forced to defend their caring role.

One specific example of organisational change, considered in an earlier part of this book, which, according to Clifford (1995), illustrates the difficulty in laying claim to caring as unique – or even central – to nursing, is the increase in numbers of support workers as part of the larger skill mix. Clifford (1995) questions whether, when these support staff are the direct care givers, albeit under the direction of qualified practitioners, nurses can claim to be more than 'carers by proxy'. As with the situation where family or friends are caring directly for dependants, how can caring, thus delegated, be described as a unique function of nursing?

But if these commentators see a very real danger of nursing today being subservient to the organisation, as perhaps it was to the medical profession in the past, there exist others who would dispute this, or at least credit nursing with an ability to transcend organisational constraints. Savage (1995), in a study of the nurse–patient relationship, sought specifically to focus on the organisational context of practice, noting that previous such research has tended to overlook this. Her findings, following one year studying two medical–surgical wards with contrasting ways of working (one a nursing development unit practising primary nursing, the other operating a less formalised patient allocation system) led her to conclude that there was little difference between the wards in the nurses' views of care, and that more important to practice than the organisational mode were the local conditions in terms of staffing levels, staff support and such like. Although the hospital ward was seen to be a bounded area, representing nurses' and patients' symbolic space within which caring actions were organised, these boundaries were seen to dissolve when nurses were giving personal care. Savage (1995) suggests here that nurses can manipulate the context, for instance by redrawing the boundaries between the public and private areas of practice.

The study by Smith (1992) of emotional labour makes much the same point. Although Smith spends time describing the setting for her research, also in a British teaching hospital, she concludes that it is not so much the setting that provides the conditions which allow for the 'emotion' part of nursing work, but individual nurses' skills which enable recognition of when it is needed in particular situations, and the ward sister who 'sets the emotional agenda' through her leadership style.

It would seem, then, that although nurses do not have the absolute freedom to practise 'caring' in its idealised form within given organisational structures, there may be ways in which the goals of such care can be achieved by the manipulation of contexts at the more local levels and, as such, maintain a nursing practice which harmonises with its philosophy to an acceptable degree. The final question is, what influence does the overarching health policy context bring to bear, within which these local organisational modes operate and which may not be so amenable to manipulation?

Health policy and political context

Health care (and therefore nursing) is a political issue and so inevitably affected by a government's health policy. However, within this bald and rather generalised statement lie a number of sub-issues which determine how this relationship may work out in practice. Three broad areas will be considered here in relation to British health policy of the 1990s: first, the extent to which nurses themselves are involved in influencing the political agenda; secondly, the nature of the link between policy ideals and their implementation, and how nurses mediate this process; thirdly, the place of nurse education as a policy and professional interest.

Cox (1993) suggests that nurses should fulfil their responsibility as the major caring profession by using their political influence and leadership potential. However, there is considerable feeling among commentators that they have singularly failed here. Tattam & Thompson (1993) observe that, while there is certainly more open debate nowadays, both about the image of nursing in general and about political issues which affect nursing (which, they say, would have been 'treasonable' a decade ago), nurses have, in fact, contributed to the process of making themselves invisible and need, instead, to effectively communicate the importance of nursing work.

This invisibility and passivity is also observed by Savage (1995), who attributes this to the way in which, in the climate of the current British National Health Service (NHS) reforms, with their emphasis on efficiency and outcome, nursing skills – less easily measured – tend to be down-played. Smith (1992), Brykczynska (1993) and Clifford (1995) all make a similar point in acknowledging the precedence of economic concerns over nursing values, especially the 'expressive' elements of care.

And yet, there is also something of a paradox noted by observers with regard to health policy reforms, which, on the face of it, might seem to be moving in harmony with nursing priorities. Tattam & Thompson (1993) cite the government's 'named nurse' initiative as likely to encourage the move to primary nursing, while Savage (1995) mentions the Patients' Charter (DoH 1992), the 'Griffiths' reorganisation (DHSS 1983) and government funding of Nursing Development Units (NDUs) in the same light. In fact, Savage detected the nature of care, as put forward in government and Audit Commission documents, to be very much in tune with what she observed in one of the wards of her research. The problem which, according to Savage, hinders the development of nursing along these lines is that, running in tandem with these facilitative directives, are pressures to engage in competing initiatives, such as the 'skill mix' issue, designed to cut cost and make services more attractive to purchasers.

Savage (1995) sees this situation as far from unique to her research. She describes a situation where nurses everywhere are being exhorted to develop good practice while being caught between two opposing views of health care. On the one hand is the rhetoric which makes health care consumers paramount and reflects the ethos of the 'new nursing'; on the other hand is the government desire to transform the NHS into an internal market, steered by cost effectiveness and, perhaps, reflecting the older, task orientation of nursing. Like Tattam & Thompson (1993) therefore, Savage questions the motives behind policy initiatives such as the 'named nurse', seeing this as being very much a secondary, 'PR' issue to a government more concerned with cutting waiting lists and other cost-effective out-comes. Such tensions, she believes, created by these opposing policy thrusts, have, arguably, always existed where a gulf occurs between what is wanted and what can be resourced. In the past this was mitigated by the goodwill of staff working within an inefficient service; now the push towards efficiency is giving rise to stress among nurses and a situation where initiatives such as the Patients' Charter become merely top–down directives disguising more pressing governmental priorities.

Whether or not one agrees with this analysis, speculation is likely to continue with regard to the overall effect of the market economy on the health professions. Smith (1992) comments that it would be interesting to speculate as to whether the privatisation of the NHS will lead to a commercialisation of nurses' emotional labour in the private health industry, while Titmuss, as long ago as 1970, was questioning whether medical (and, by analogy, nursing) care could be seen as a consumer good indistinguishable from other such goods in a private economic market

(Titmuss 1970). If Campbell's (1984) view that there can be no synthesis between the personal and the political holds good (on the grounds that politics is alien to caring), then the present and future status of nursing does, perhaps, look marginal and bleak.

Yet there is another issue at stake here, and that concerns whether there is a linear relationship between policy as ideals and policy as it is implemented. This, again, could amount to a double-edged sword. On the one hand is the view as put forward by Cox (1993) with reference to the NHS and Community Care Act, 1990, that, though the community care reforms were based on humane and idealistic motives, their implementation has been fraught with problems and they therefore have not lived up to these ideals. On the other hand there is the argument put forward by Lipsky (1980) that what he calls 'street level bureaucrats', that is professionals working 'at the sharp end', have a considerable amount of discretion as they interpret policy and are, therefore, not entirely without influence in the exercise of their professional practice.

There must certainly be an element of truth in both these viewpoints. There is, for instance, evidence from research that community nurses acting as case managers, in the wake of community care implementation, perceived the philosophy behind case management to be totally positive from a nursing perspective, even though the means to introducing it (largely 'top–down') left much to be desired (Bergen 1995). Even Lipsky (1980) implicitly recognises that policy intent and policy implementation may not match when he comments that, whereas all policy reformers are supportive of policy ideals, it is a 'myth of service altruism' (p.21) that public institutions and government policy can respond fully to the needs of citizens, and that the requirements of the state and the interests of those citizens are necessarily congruent.

Lipsky's (1980) well-developed theory about street level bureaucrats, however, may offer hope to professionals who feel powerless in the face of policy directives. Lipsky theorises that 'street level bureaucrats exercise discretion to such an extent that they are not easily affected by policy articulation from above' (Lipsky, 1980, p.119). In a sense they are able to 'become' public policies in themselves, because policy, as laid out in guidelines, is necessarily vague and often ambiguous, and also because such professionals (and here he includes teachers, the police and judges, as well as nurses) work largely autonomously in practice.

Not that Lipsky (1980) implies this is an easy undertaking. Indeed, he acknowledges that for street level bureaucrats 'the very nature of their work prevents them from coming even close to the ideal conception of their jobs' (p. xiii). The constraints of the real-life context, in the form of large caseloads or classes, inadequate resources, the unpredictability of clients and uncertain conditions, defeat the aspiration of many service workers. Moreover, he argues, 'to deliver street level policy through bureaucracy is to embrace a contradiction' (p.21); ideally, and by training, these professionals respond to the individual needs of the people they serve, but because of the bureaucratic structure within which they operate, they are constrained to deal with clients on a detached, mass basis. Any personalised human interaction must be delivered on a discretionary basis, and it is in this discretionary element of practice that any residuum of power to interpret policy resides. Again, there is empirical evidence to suggest this may be applicable to nursing practice; a number of the community nurse case managers referred to above suggested that practices often straddled official community care implementation. It was their own professional decision-making, rather than policy directives, which dictated the adoption of certain models of care for certain clients (Bergen 1995).

The final issue in the policy arena, although perhaps less immediate than the considerations addressed above, is that of nurse education, since this is to a certain extent governed by political interests which again may either promote or inhibit professionally defined practice. Both Perry (1993) and Tattam & Thompson (1993) decipher a certain degree of divergence here between the way nurse academics are mapping out educational preparation, and the way government thinking appears to be heading. Thus, while nurses are seeking a more academic basis to their learning, government policy of the 1990s is attempting to reform teacher and social work education by re-introducing the more traditional apprenticeship-style, practical emphasis.

On the other hand, teaching has been described as a political activity in itself (Pendleton 1993), implying that, whatever structures may be imposed from without, nurse educators may still retain some power with regard to content; thus ideals may, at least, be passed on. However, again one must question how reflective of nursing reality this is if divorced from the practice context. The nature of clinical support and educational resources – or lack of them – actually 'tells' students something about their own value and the values of the profession of which they are part. As Brykczynska (1993) notes, an effective power base in nursing education is formed where academics and practitioners (and, hopefully, policy makers) work together.

Conclusion: nursing – the reality

This chapter has argued that any analysis of nursing as caring cannot be made in isolation from the real world of nursing practice, which itself is influenced by a number of changing contexts. It has been suggested that the contexts chosen here for consideration – historical, social, organisational and political – must inevitably influence practice to some degree, but, at the same time, nurses are not without the ability, within any of these, to forge a reality which is representative of their practice ideals. It has also been argued that there is, perhaps, no single reality in such a diverse occupation, nor should one be sought; what is deemed appropriate in one setting or in one specialism may be of less import in another. What is clear is that nurses, both individually and corporately, must develop confidence to exert their influence in society, in management and in the policy making arena so that they are able to take what is facilitative and change what is detrimental to care in any given context.

References

Benner, P. & Wrubel, J. (1989) *The Primacy of Caring: Stress and Coping in Health and Illness.* Addison-Wesley, California.

Bergen, A. (1995) *A study to identify the current and potential relevance and value of case management to community nursing.* The Queen's Nursing Institute, London.

Bignold, S., Cribb, A. & Ball, S. (1995) Befriending the family: an exploration of a nurse–client relationship. *Health & Social Care in the Community,* 3, 173–80.

Bradshaw, A. (1995) What are nurses doing to patients? A review of theories of nursing past and present. *Journal of Clinical Nursing,* 4, 81–92.

Brykczynska, G. (1993) Nursing values: nightmares and nonsense. In: *Nursing: its Hidden Agendas,* (eds M. Jolley & G. Brykczynska). Edward Arnold, London.

Campbell, A.V. (1984) *Moderated love: a theology of medical care.* SPCK, London.

Clifford, C. (1995) Caring: fitting the concept to nursing practice. *Journal of Clinical Nursing,* 4, 37–41.

Cox, C. (1993) Closing thoughts on hidden agendas – an epilogue. In: *Nursing: its Hidden Agendas,* (eds M. Jolley & G. Brykczynska). Edward Arnold, London.

Department of Health (1992) *The Patient's Charter.* HMSO, London.

DHSS (Department of Health & Social Security) (1983) *NHS Management Inquiry.* HMSO, London.

Fealy, G.M. (1995) Professional caring: the moral dimension. *Journal of Advanced Nursing,* 22, 1135–40.

Jolley, M. (1993) Out of the past. In *Nursing: its Hidden Agendas,* (eds M. Jolley & G. Brykczynska). Edward Arnold, London.

Lawler, J. (1991) *Behind the Screens: Nursing, Somology and the Problem of the Body.* Churchill-Livingstone, Melbourne, Australia.

Lea, A. & Watson, R. (1996) Caring research and concepts: a selected review of the literature. *Journal of Clinical Nursing,* 5, 71–77.

Lipsky, M. (1980) *Street Level Bureaucracy: Dilemmas of the Individual in Public Services.* Russell Sage Foundation, New York.

Melia, K. (1987) *Learning and Working: the Occupational Socialization of Nurses.* Tavistock, London.

Miers, M. (1996) Do they mean us? *Nursing Standard,* **10**(15), 20–21.

Nursing Standard (1996) News. *Nursing Standard,* **11**(16), 7.

Pendleton, S. (1993) Hidden curricula in nursing education. In *Nursing: its Hidden Agendas,* (eds M. Jolley & G. Brykczynska). Edward Arnold, London.

Perry, A. (1993) A sociologist's view: the handmaiden's theory. In *Nursing: its Hidden Agendas,* (eds M. Jolley & G. Brykczynska). Edward Arnold, London.

Savage, J. (1995) *Nursing Intimacy: an Ethnographic Approach to Nurse–patient Interaction.* Scutari Press, London.

Smith, P. (1992) *The Emotional Labour of Nursing: How Nurses Care.* Macmillan, Basingstoke.

Tattam, A. & Thompson, M. (1993) Political influences in nursing. In *Nursing: its Hidden Agendas,* (eds M. Jolley & G. Brykczynska). Edward Arnold, London.

Titmuss, R.M. (1970) *The Gift Relationship: from Human Blood to Social Policy.* Allen & Unwin, London.

Wade, S. (1995) Partnership in care: a critical review. *Nursing Standard,* **9**(48), 29–32.

Warelow, P.J. (1996) Is caring the ethical ideal? *Journal of Advanced Nursing,* 24, 655–61.

Webb, C. (1996) Caring, curing, coping: towards an integrated model. *Journal of Advanced Nursing,* 32, 960–68.

9 Opportunities in a Managerial Age

Margaret Edwards and Nicholas Hale

Introduction

This book opened by noting the insistent pace of change as the twentieth century draws to a close. The gradual movement towards managerialism appears as an underlying theme, albeit one peppered with spasmodic lurches in one direction or another. Emerging similarities between visions of 'new professionalism' and 'new management' were identified at the start, but the practicalities of implementing real change within complex organisational systems have been acknowledged. The other chapters have continued the themes introduced in the initial analysis. The professional commitment of nurses to caring as a therapeutic endeavour has been acknowledged and criticised. Likewise, problems stemming from a managerial commitment to organisational efficiency have been identified, yet the need to ensure a quality service overall has been accepted.

This final chapter is being written as the Labour Government, elected in May 1997, has issued its proposals for reforming the National Health Service (DoH 1997). By its own admission the Government has not sought to overhaul the major reforms implemented through the NHS and Community Care Act 1990. Rather, it has attempted to build on the perceived successes of those reforms while removing what it considered to be the divisive structure of the internal market. Recurring throughout the new white paper are ideas of integration, co-operation and the search for a 'third way' to unify formerly competing ideas and factions in working towards a shared goal of creating a 'New NHS' that will be modern and dependable (DoH 1997).

Cynically, these intentions might be regarded as a political manoeuvre that aims to please everyone but which may succeed only in papering over the real problems and power bases that pertain within the health service. However, they offer a useful opportunity to illustrate the general thrust of this text, which has aimed to shed light on a way for nursing to articulate its particular contribution to human well-being. The potential, highlighted at the outset, of integrating the common vision and ideals of new professionalism and new managerialism in a shared agenda gave way to a consideration of the practicalities of working under different organisational imperatives. Picking up on those practical insights, this chapter will use the proposals for a 'New NHS' to return to the integrating vision set out at the start. Finally, the chapter and book will conclude by stressing the important role of nursing research in developing an evidence base to support contentions about the contribution that nursing can make to society.

The 'New NHS'

Economy and organisation

The NHS is reported to cost the nation £1000 a second (DoH 1997) and represents an enormous drain on the national exchequer. It is therefore unlikely that any government will ever allow this costly organisation to drift again, or be pulled hither and thither by the whims and aspirations of professionals as was the perceived case during the period when consensus management was the organisational method. Yet ostensibly the white paper appears to be devolving responsibility for the management of resources to clinicians working in primary care, particularly general medical practitioners (GPs).

Monies to finance the new organisational changes will reportedly flow in part from the reduction in administration costs that were incurred as a result of the internal market. As Wells reports in Chapter 4, the number of managers proliferated following the 1990 reforms as the annual round of contracting required their particular skills. Whether the health service is about to witness the fall from grace of the professional manager has yet to be seen, but the bureaucracy of the internal market is a key target for reform and management costs will be capped. The new proposals suggest that it will be through clinician to clinician partnership that service agreements aimed at securing health gain will be focused.

Primary care lead

In line with previous policy, the 'New NHS' will look to general practice to be the hub of the Health Service. Studies in the USA and across a number of European countries (Starfield 1992, 1994) have shown a consistent relationship between the availability of primary care physicians and health levels as assessed by age-adjusted and standardised overall mortality, mortality associated with cancer and heart disease, neonatal mortality and life expectancy – even after controlling for the effect of urban/rural differences, poverty rates, education and lifestyle, etc. Findings from these studies also suggest that countries where health systems are more orientated towards primary care achieve better health levels, higher satisfaction with health services among their populations and lower costs of services.

Such evidence explains why health care policy in the UK has increasingly focused on primary care as the heart of the health care system. The 1991–2 National Morbidity Study found that in Great Britain 78% of the population consulted their GP at least once annually (McCormack *et al.* 1995). General practice would therefore seem to be a logical fulcrum around which to base health care services. Recent policy initiatives from the Department of Health (DoH 1996a, 1996b) have tended to view primary health care as care delivered or co-ordinated by GPs. The 'New NHS' proposals stress the inclusion of community nurses and other professionals in primary care; despite this, the plans are widely interpreted as being mainly aimed at putting GPs in the lead.

Under the proposed changes the government aims to build on some of the benefits that have accrued from the reforms while altering the divisive nature inherent in an organisational arrangement that produced a two-tier system. Under GP fundholding some patients obtained earlier and greater access to treatment than others regardless of clinical need (DoH 1997). It is hoped that the perceived successes of fundholding and the other models of GP commissioning in sharpening the responses of some hospital services and extending the range of provision available in their own surgeries will continue under the proposed system of Primary Care Groups (PCGs).

Commissioning for health

It is envisaged that groups of GPs in a locality will play a key role in PCGs that will commission health services. To some extent, these will build on and develop locality commissioning schemes, where groups of GPs worked together to plan and commission services, and total purchasing projects where GPs worked outside fundholding to purchase hospital and community health services. However, there is a clear determination to avoid simply adding to 'GP power'. In the transition towards PCGs, decision-making processes are intended to involve a wide range of health service professionals as well as public and voluntary organisations. Emphasising that discussions must be genuinely open, the guidance insists that there should be no presumption that unilateral proposals from health authorities, GPs or NHS trusts will necessarily be the basis for PCGs (NHSE 1998a, b).

Health authorities will gradually relinquish their overall commissioning function to PCGs who, over time, could become free standing bodies (Primary Care Trusts), accountable to the health authority but responsible for the provision of community services for their population. There would be the possibility for PCGs to assume financial responsibility for both hospital and community services. These PCGs will cover a population of about 100 000 represented on 50 or so general practice lists, although there is flexibility depending on local circumstances. Groups are required to have a governing body that includes community nurses and social services; they are charged with working within the local health improvement programme.

As their local commissioning functions are absorbed by PCGs, health authorities will develop a wider strategic role, developing public health in collaboration across health and social services. Each health authority will lead the drawing up of a Health Improvement Programme (HImP) in consultation with primary care groups, NHS trusts (including acute hospital trusts, specialist mental health and learning disability services) and social services. The HImP will represent the business plan for each health authority, but it is envisaged that it must demonstrate how the health of the local population will be enhanced, drawing on public health insights.

The white paper (DoH 1997) is explicit in requiring health authorities, PCGs and trusts to work intersectorally with other agencies, including local authorities, to draw up the Health Improvement Programmes for the population they cover. The emphasis on primary care and the commissioning power of the PCGs is likely to affect considerably the nature of these plans, which has implications not only for community nurses but also for those working in acute hospitals and within specialist mental health and learning disability services.

Management and the professions

The consultation document on public health (DoH 1998) is particularly explicit in emphasising the multidisciplinary and multi-agency nature of this work, although no financial accountability exists beyond the immediate remit of clinical services provided by the NHS. The use of integrating frameworks in those public health proposals (DoH 1998) and for assessing performance within the 'New NHS' (NHSE 1998b) implies a major organisational shift from an old-style, goal-directed bureaucracy towards the flexibility inherent in organisations based on holographic principles (see Chapter 1 of this book and Morgan and Ramirez 1983). This shift is represented, too, in the introduction of 'clinical governance', which is intended to bring the skills of health care professionals to bear on the traditional managerial problems of ensuring efficiency, effectiveness and quality assurance across the organisation of the health service.

Through the 1970s and 1980s nursing was moving towards a more holistic approach to work organisation as it espoused the notion of primary nursing. This approach to work could be equated with new-wave management thought. Within this ideology can be found the terms post-Fordist, post-modern and post-bureaucratic. These approaches have been dominant in managerial thought since the work of McGregor (1960), but according to some commentators have at best received a sceptical reception within the NHS (Pollitt 1993). The belief within these approaches to organisational form is that in the absence of cohesive mechanisms, productivity is best achieved not through compliance or passive accommodation but by moving towards self-control. Jobs are broadly defined with less central control and more autonomous decision-making.

Reflecting the philosophy of the central administration, the 'New NHS' white paper is eclectic in its approach and appears at first reading to contain elements of both the Fordist and post-Fordist approaches to management (Hoggett 1996) which are discussed in Chapter 5. Under the new arrangements, clinicians within the Primary Care Groups will be given the opportunities to commission the services that they deem necessary for their locality. This arrangement appears distinctly post-Fordist in that clinicians will be allowed to shape the services which they provide and indeed have financial responsibility for these. However, the changes mean that GP budgets will effectively be subject to direct control for the first time since the start of the NHS.

The burning question for nursing is how it will fare under a system that is devolving decision-making for the delivery of care to clinicians. They are the most numerous group included in the given definition of 'health professionals who are directly involved in the care and treatment of patients, for example, nurses, doctors, therapists, midwives' (DoH 1997). Does this mean the millennium will represent the golden age for nursing when the aspirations of the occupation will finally find expression? A closer examination of the implications for nursing stemming from the proposed changes may go some way to answering this question.

Nursing implications

Strategic involvement

The present government has placed an emphasis on public health, and PCGs will need to adopt this perspective when commissioning local services. Yet GPs have shown little appetite for public health or health promotion (Russell 1994). While recognising the effects of poverty and lifestyle on health they have perceived public health to lie outside their spheres of activity, which have consisted in providing secondary preventive medical services. When the GP contract of 1990 required that GPs engage with health promotion activities, an army of practice nurses was imported (Atkin & Hirst 1994).

As the demand on GPs to provide secondary preventive care for their patients is unlikely to decrease, opportunities may arise for community nurses to discharge the public health functions required under the new white paper, particularly with respect to local needs assessment and intersectoral working. For nurses, a best case scenario would be that in which nurses work in partnership with GPs to assess local health needs (not just medical needs) and are influential players in the commissioning process of the PCGs. The worst case would be that of a powerful group of GPs dominating a PCG, simply paying lip service to the involvement of nurses and commissioning only services that meet the needs of secondary preventive medical care.

Some nurses envisage a turf war between GPs and nurses and history tells us that medicine is more likely to be the winner in any such conflict; government agreement that doctors will always be in a majority and have the right to choose a chairman from among their number is an early illustration of this (NHSE 1998c). Even so, many nurses have expressed delight at the opportunities offered within the white paper, while recognising that in order to grasp the possibilities on offer nurses are likely to need to develop skills to enable them to be full players in commissioning and the management of PCGs (Rowe 1998). Anecdotally the reaction of GPs to the involvement of nurses in primary care groups appears mixed, with some being dismissive and scornful and others welcoming the idea wholeheartedly.

As Wells notes in Chapter 4, nurses historically have displayed a certain distaste for management. This may have been associated with the major difficulty that being involved in any strategic planning or taking on responsibility at an organisational level has, hitherto, meant leaving clinical practice. However, beyond the rhetoric it is unknown how much real appetite there is among practising nurses for the strategic involvement required in the brave new world of PCGs.

Under the 1990 reforms, the desire to grasp the nettle was not universal among GPs themselves, who did not subscribe wholeheartedly to fund-holding (Duggan 1995) This reticence has been acknowledged by the government and PCGs will be able to choose the level at which they wish to operate, at least initially. The ultimate aim is for PCGs to assume financial responsibility for the commissioning of both hospital and community services. This level of responsibility and control seems to signal a move to post-Fordist managerial approaches. The degree of autonomy being afforded to the PCGs may well appear attractive to the professions and in particular to doctors who were the particular target for control under the previous administration (DoH 1989).

However, while increased responsibility for the management of resources will be devolved to clinicians working in primary care, the proposals also mean that general practitioner budgets will effectively be cost-limited for the first time since the start of the NHS. Furthermore, the principles embedded in the white paper and guidance about the process of setting up the PCGs (DoH 1997, NHSE 1998a) do not reflect the old-fashioned professional notions of exclusiveness, unique knowledge and independent autonomous actions set out in Chapter 1 of this book. Rather, they resemble Davies' (1995) new vision of professionalism, emphasising interdependent decision-making, collective responsibility and patient involvement. The extent to which traditional power patterns will prevail remains an open question at present, but the proposals offer at least the potential for the first steps to be taken towards a real change in organisational approach.

Substitution and skill mix

Notwithstanding Cowley's assertion in Chapter 1 that nursing is less dependent on medicine in the community than in hospitals, the notion of the primary health care team shows that nursing has been perceived as a medical activity. Although the concept of the primary health care team was first advanced in the early 1920s (MoH 1920), it was really only from the late 1960s onwards, following the Report of the Royal Commission on Medical Education (1968), that the attachment of nurses to general practices gained momentum.

The report advocated group practices and argued that GPs needed to delegate a variety of tasks to colleagues in other professions. The report was unambiguous in its view that the GP would be the leader of any team of health care professionals involved in primary care. Nurses and health visitors were seen as becoming integral members of *medical* practice. Many of the tensions within primary health care teams have stemmed from this belief. There have been particular tensions between GPs and health visitors, the latter having their origins within the nineteenth century public health movements and traditionally espousing a more psychosocial model of care (Edwards 1998). Indeed, some would argue that the emphasis on facilitation and public health rather than the direct delivery of care to patients with specified needs, means that health visiting sits uneasily within a primary care nursing framework (Mackereth 1996, Symonds 1997).

It is clear, therefore, that the advent of the PCGs represents both threats and opportunities. The white paper stresses that nurses and community nurses in particular have a significant role to play, particularly in contributing to the assessment of need required for the commissioning of services that will make up the Health Improvement Programme. Yet the lead role given to GPs brings threats to those community nurses who, under fundholding, baulked at the prospect of direct employment by general practitioners fearing that their work would be controlled by doctors and that they would be forced to work to a purely medical model.

What may be an unpalatable fact for the nursing profession, but what appears to be none the less the case, is that nurses may be valuable to governments precisely because they are able to provide safe substitution for many areas of medical practice. Successful evaluations of disease-specific nurse specialist posts only go to prove the point (Hamilton *et al.* 1995). Many of the professions allied to medicine, who arguably have less flexibility to substitute for medicine, have not figured prominently in the white paper and have expressed concern about the nature of the proposed changes (Gulland 1998). Substituting for medicine may in fact be a particular strength and a useful bargaining point for nursing, though many nurses would probably not agree (Bradshaw 1998).

It has already been noted in relation to changes in medical work and recruitment that there is a domino effect within the health service and changes to the professional status of doctors will in turn affect that of nurses. These demographics are providing changes and opportunities for community nurses in previously uncharted waters. The Primary Care Act pilots (NHSE 1997), which allow nurse-led initiatives, could be seen as opportunities to provide medical services in areas like London where there is a severe GP recruitment and retention problem.

The NHS (Primary Care) Act 1997 included provision for the piloting of innovative methods of delivering primary care services, including the opportunity for nurses to lead some of these pilots. In a complete reversal of the usual status quo, the legislation enables nurses in these pilot sites to employ medical practitioners when medical input is required (DoH 1996a). Among the ten nurse-led sites funded to commence in 1998, there are three pilots in which nurse practitioners will deliver the full range of personal medical services, referring to a partner general medical practitioner if required. What the Victorian surgeons, shuddering at the thought of nurses testing urine, would have made of this can only be a case for speculation. However, shortfalls in medical recruitment to general practice (particularly in the inner cities), reductions in hospital doctors' working hours together with the enormous strides made by nursing over the last century, are making such innovations possible.

Yet it has already been noted in an earlier chapter that nursing itself is facing a shortfall in recruitment and the pressures to relieve the medical workload are impinging on other areas of work that many nurses have felt were more legitimately theirs. Downward pressure appears to be relegating traditional areas of nursing work to health care assistants. Allocating tasks to health care assistants seems to signal a return to Fordist methods of work organisation, where production is broken down into simpler tasks and is co-ordinated by rules implemented by a centralised management. Jobs are simplified in the process and work can be done by cheaper, less skilled and less flexible workers (Walby *et al.* 1994). Taking blood is an example of this. In hospitals it used to be the work of junior doctors and in the community of district nurses and GPs. The trend has been in hospital to employ specially trained phlebotomists, and in some GP surgeries receptionists have been trained to take blood to allow practice nurses to devote more time to health promotion and disease management clinics.

The result for the patient in the GP surgery is less waiting time, and this is the important issue. A traditional professional perspective would insist on regulation – as in the days when nurses were expected to be 'certificated' prior to carrying out the so-called extended role of venepuncture – to be sure that the procedure could be carried out correctly. A traditional management perspective would demand that every step of a procedure is separately and strictly controlled with no built-in flexibility for the workers concerned. However, the question of whether or not work is fragmented or adequately carried out should be assessed, not from the perspective of the practitioners (whether doctors or nurses), but from the point of view of the person on the receiving end of the practice. The potential to import a 'holistic focus' to the work by emphasising the centrality of patients is considered further below.

Changing patterns of care

The intention to move even more services to the primary care setting is apparent in the white paper, changing the nature of work for both community and acute hospital nurses. The latter are unlikely to see a reduction in patient throughput, but even shorter hospital stays for acute episodes are more likely to be the order of the day. While the pace of change may accelerate, new patterns of care have evolved in recent years to take account of changing needs and the wish to improve the overall co-ordination of service delivery. Two examples are particularly relevant for the purposes of this chapter, as they demonstrate the potential for enhancing patient experience by developing new organisational arrangements for the delivery of nursing care.

First, community nurses will be caring for ever more patients who have greater levels of acute illness than previously (CSAG 1997). Hospital at home schemes have proliferated and evaluations have shown that outcomes for patients have not been compromised, though the work of some schemes is thought to have impacted significantly on the work of other community agencies and may not have suited all patients (Fulop *et al.* 1997). Most of the schemes reported in the literature have been nurse led and a striking feature of many of the schemes is the use of support workers working with district nurses to sustain the patient at home. Many of the schemes involve enhanced nursing care at home for elderly patients, and the effects of an ageing population have already been felt in community nursing, particularly as numbers of district nurses have been falling over the years (CSAG 1997).

The second example of organisational innovation – patient focused care – has developed in institutional settings. PFC, or hospital process re-engineering as it has sometimes been called (Green 1994), could loosely be described as a framework for care delivery where the patient pathway is key and needs are met by multiskilled, cross-trained professionals. This framework can minimise what management consultants Booz-Allen and Hamilton (1990) refer to as 'system idle time' (where getting ready for action, organising the action to take place at an appropriate time and documenting action is taking much longer than the action itself), thus hastening the patient's pathway through the system.

In the literature, the patient focused care framework appears to consist of a number of components, each of which impact on professional work. Not all these identified components will necessarily exist together, as implementation of patient focused care in hospitals appears to be heavily influenced by the culture of the host organisation (Pollitt 1996). The components of patient focused care include among others, decentralised services, multiskilled staff, cross training, multidisciplinary care protocols, clinical pathways, minimisation of patient movement, staff empowerment and hospitals organised around a product line, and finally transparent quality control. Patient focused care is clearly an approach that accords with the intentions of 'the New NHS' (DoH 1997).

An idealised vision of the PFC team is a post-Fordist team of empowered multiskilled individuals (Walby *et al.* 1994). Skills present in the team are determined by an analysis of the needs of patients (Manthey 1994). This is an optimistic vision where teams are made up of workers with enriched jobs that enable them to meet the majority of patients' needs without complex, labour intensive referrals. This kind of vision would not sit uncomfortably with primary nursing, although within this organisation of nursing work the person meeting the patients' needs is predominantly a highly trained qualified nurse. In primary nursing the patient is placed at the centre as in the patient focused care framework but, in its quest for the holy grail of self definition and liberation from subservience to medicine, nursing has often failed to take a multidisciplinary approach.

It is arguable therefore whether primary nursing can be said to be truly patient centred as the needs of the patient are defined in terms of nursing, and quality defined in terms of nursing outcomes, although some might argue that these do not or should not differ from patient outcomes. Professional preoccupations (Robinson 1994) and interprofessional conflict (Carpenter 1995) have been said to blur the understanding of patient need within existing multidisciplinary care team organisation. Buchan (1995) argues that compartmentalised, functional over-specialisation and custom and practice create inefficiencies and under use of resources. The PFC team would be one where traditional boundaries shift to meet the needs of patients in modern health care settings. In the community setting, integrated nursing teams of health visitors, district nurses and practice nurses are becoming the preferred configurations (at least of managers).

Porter-O'Grady (1993) has discussed the radical 're-professionalisation' of care teams where the role of professional activity is unquestioned but professional boundaries are restructured. However, it is exactly this notion of functional flexibility that creates so many problems for nurses. The Royal College of Nursing (RCN 1992) has adopted a more pessimistic and professionally defensive stance towards PFC, viewing it as a vehicle for de-professionalisation. Functional flexibility in its view is translated, not as extending the competence of nurses, but as developing the role of an unqualified, non-professional generic health care worker.

In its analysis such numerically as well as functionally flexible workers become a receptacle for those high-volume low complexity jobs carried out by the professional occupational groupings (RCN 1992). The relegation of such tasks to unqualified workers fails to take account of the distinction between technical and intellectual aspects of care activities (Braithewaite 1995) and marks a return to task orientation. For McMahon (1991) the process of functional specialisation has led to an erosion of the nurse's therapeutic impact on care for patients. There is, however, evidence that with appropriate leadership unqualified staff can deliver therapeutic care to patients (Thomas 1992).

Again, it seems that a shift is needed, so that the emphasis is on whether the person on the receiving end of professional care perceives the experience as holistic, and whether the end result is a gain in health. This approach could demonstrate the potential benefit of having professional nurses who co-ordinate, manage and organise the delivery of care; although, in a multidisciplinary age it must be acknowledged that sometimes that role might fall more appropriately to an occupational therapist, medical practitioner or other professional. This is a clear and deliberate change in emphasis from the professional role to which nursing has long aspired.

Changing emphasis

It is clear that insistence that all nursing activities must be carried out by registered nurses is no longer sustainable, and the deliberations in this book have led us to question whether it is necessarily always desirable. It remains equally clear that nursing has a significant and important contribution to make to the welfare of the population it serves and the shift proposed in this chapter should not be interpreted as casting any doubt on our collective belief in the value of nursing. However, questions about how nursing is to be delivered and the means of its organisation appear more important than continuing to strive towards either managerial or professionalising ideals that, in themselves, are falling into disrepute.

Caring ideals

It would probably not be useful to rehearse again the issues around the therapeutic value of nursing. However, certain questions do need to be asked if nursing can only define itself through a self-styled monopoly of caring when organisational changes beyond the control of the profession mean that at worst that function must be relinquished and at best delegated to unqualified staff.

The first question concerns those periods in the history of nursing where task allocation was acknowledged unashamedly as the method of nursing work. How did nursing sustain the support and admiration of the public before the advent of primary nursing? The esteem that the nursing profession enjoys preceded its dalliance with new organisational forms. As Morrison and Cowley point out in Chapter 2, the public appreciate the technical skills of nurses and do require them to have a particular approach. In those studies where the public rated most highly the technical skills of nurses, the requirement to have a caring approach may have preceded this response as a cultural given that did not need expression. Even so, ensuring sufficient variety of skills within a nursing team delivering care, and ensuring that the team leader is able to exercise adequate control over delegated activities, is a viable alternative to insisting that only registered nurses have the knowledge and skills required to carry out caring functions.

A key question is whether humanistic approaches and caring attitudes can be delegated to or instilled in generic support workers who will be delivering a large proportion of basic care to patients. There is certainly enough evidence to support the argument that quality of leadership and unit philosophies are influential in the way that ancillary staff work. Also key is whether under a patient focused system, the qualified nurse will in fact be directing generic support workers or whether this group will evolve into a separate occupational group as the Royal College of Nursing fear. The answer may well lie with nurses themselves as to whether they are prepared to embrace these workers within the nursing team and whether professional organisations such as the RCN are prepared to admit them to their ranks.

The issue of quality

Returning to the main analysis of a framework for patient focused care and the white paper, one of the most striking features in both is an emphasis on quality. The quality debate is itself part of the general approach to the restructuring of the public sector in the UK. The emergence of quality into the discourse of the NHS is generally marked by the publication of an earlier white paper *Working for Patients* (DoH 1989) and has been perceived as a managerial attempt to control expenditure in a uniquely complex organisation. What in fact emerged from managerial attempts to get quality onto the agenda was the hijacking of quality by the varying professional groups.

Pollitt (1993) puts this situation succinctly when he says that the issue of quality was quickly divided up along tribal lines. As a result the concept of quality has remained elusive between and within professional boundaries. Nursing writing in this area is exemplified by Bond and Thomas (1991) searching for outcomes that are specific to nursing. Discussion of nurse specific outcomes is often linked to the anxiety of functional redundancy threatened by non-professional subdivision and skill substitution within nursing work. The concern to establish a link between a rich nursing skill mix and quality care can lead to a concern for mono-disciplinary audit and what Nolan (1994) calls professional defensiveness.

The 'New NHS' white paper (DoH 1997) is clear that the delivery of health care is a collective responsibility. Although the system of clinical governance is designed to emphasise the opportunity for health professionals to control their own practice, there will be a legislative requirement to collaborate across disciplines and agencies and ultimate accountability falls to the chief executive of the organisation. Health Improvement Plans will be subjected to an unprecedented level of scrutiny from the centre in an attempt to control quality. While the specifications and guidance are, so far, being kept to a critical minimum, the control is a clear and substantial counterpoint to the apparent freedoms afforded to clinicians in their commissioning decisions. This may be seen as an attempt to check professional power, or to develop an organisation that promotes the kind of shared responsibility and 'double loop learning' (Argyris and Schön 1978) described in Chapter 1.

Nursing and the use of clinical guidelines

The 'New NHS' contains an unprecedented number of mechanisms for controlling quality within the organisation and is adopting a collective approach to the delivery of a common service product. More than ever before, the emphasis will be on outcomes and evidence of effectiveness rather than process. Clinical guidelines have been welcomed by practitioners who do not have time to read the necessary literature on every area of care that must be delivered. The problem is that there is so little hard evidence available as yet on which to base action, which is not really acknowledged within the white paper, though clearly the work of the national institutes will be to produce more (NHSE 1998d). Hard evidence that exists is generally related to discrete medical conditions.

For nurses working in acute units where there is rapid throughput for patients with single pathology, the use of protocols may ease the process of decision-making and for all nurses may afford some protection against consumer demands. These are first encountered by those working on the front line who do not have control of the resources. However, it is important that guidelines are utilised to enhance the effectiveness of care, as evidenced through research, and not merely as an excuse to control practitioners.

In a nationwide study of the guidelines used for health visitor prioritising of vulnerable families, none were found that met the most basic criteria of reliability or validity (Appleton 1997, Appleton & Cowley 1997). A minority were quite subjective, insensitive and potentially even less reliable than the 'unknown quantity' of individual practitioners' professional judgements. Despite this, in a third of the cases they were being used in contract setting to control practice. Many protocols for the prevention of pressure sores insist on the use of risk calculators even though these have performed badly when subjected to rigorous research scrutiny. In particular, the Waterlow risk calculator has been found to have little reliability and validity when used within district nursing as a means to determine the provision of pressure sore relieving equipment (Edwards 1995).

However, if nursing aspires to control its own practice and be valued for making a major contribution to the whole service, the evidence base for nursing interventions needs to be considerably enhanced. On paper opportunities exist at every level for nurses to influence the delivery of health care. Expert nurses with advanced research skills will need to ensure that they are involved with the Institute for Clinical Excellence and that nurses contribute significantly to the composition of the national service frameworks. A nursing contribution to clinical guidelines may help to ensure that these are in fact sensitive to the patients' need for care. The proposals encapsulated within the 'New NHS' framework make it clear that, in future, there will be no support for delivering approaches to care that are not backed by substantial research.

Where now for nursing?

The 'New NHS' white paper (DoH 1997) is explicit in its view that nurses have a significant role to play in the new organisational changes. It aims, too, to bring health care professionals into the sphere of managerial decision-making, within a far more multidisciplinary, multi-agency and co-operative organisational framework than has ever been proposed before. The extent to which these proposals will succeed can only be a matter for conjecture.

There is no automatic right to leadership in any sphere, whatever the aspirations of the professions. The certainty, then, is that nurses must earn the right to be listened to. This will not be achieved by asserting either professional rights or striving to climb managerial hierarchies, but by demonstrating the contribution to health care received by the patients and clients served by the health service as a whole. Nursing has a huge potential contribution to make; this needs to be harnessed in the most effective way to serve patients and clients. The individual, therapeutic focus of professional nursing needs to be extended to encompass responsibility for assuring overall quality by facilitating and delegating as well as delivering hands-on care. Finally, nurses need to contribute to their own knowledge base through research and raising awareness of the relevance and use of evidence based practice within multi-agency and multi-professional settings.

References

Appleton, J. (1997) Establishing the validity and reliability of clinical practice guidelines used to identify families requiring increased health visitor support. *Public Health*, 111, 107–13.

Appleton, J.V. & Cowley, S. (1997) Analysing clinical practice guidelines: a method of documentary analysis. *Journal of Advanced Nursing*, 25, 1008–17.

Argyris, C. & Schön, D. (1978) *Organisational Learning: a theory of action perspective.* Addison Wesley, Reading, Massachusetts.

Atkin, K. & Hirst, M. (1994) *Costing practice nurses: implications for primary health care.* Discussion paper 117. University of York, York.

Bond, S. & Thomas, L.H. (1991) Issues in measuring outcomes of nursing. *Journal of Advanced Nursing*, 16, 1492–1502.

Booz-Allen and Hamilton (1990) Operational restructuring the 'patient-focused hospital'. Health Care Viewpoint, London.

Bradshaw, A. (1998) Charting some challenges in the art and science of nursing. *Lancet*, 351, 438–40.

Buchan, J. (1995) Patient focus pocus. *Nursing Management*, **2**(7), 6–7.

Carpenter, J. (1995) Doctors and nurses: stereotypes and stereotype in interprofessional education. *Journal of Interprofessional Care*, **9**(2), 151–61.

CSAG (Clinical Standards Advisory Group) (1997) *Community Health Care for Elderly People.* The Stationery Office, London.

Davies, C. (1995) *Gender and the Professional Predicament of Nursing.* Open University Press, Buckingham.

DoH (Department of Health) (1989) *White Paper: Working for Patients.* The Stationery Office, London.

DoH (Department of Health) (1996a) *Primary Care: The Future – Choice and Opportunity.* The Stationery Office, London.

DoH (Department of Health) (1996b) *Primary Care: Delivering the Future.* The Stationery Office, London.

DoH (Department of Health) (1997) *The New NHS. Modern. Dependable.* Cmnd 3807. The Stationery Office, London.

DoH (Department of Health) (1998) *Our Healthier Nation.* Cmd 3852. The Stationery Office, London.

Duggan, M. (1995) *Primary Care: A Prognosis.* Institute for Public Policy Research, London.

Edwards, M. (1995) The levels of reliability and validity of the Waterlow pressure sore risk calculator. *Journal of Wound Care,* **4**(8), 373–8.

Edwards, M. (1998) Primary health care. In: *Nursing Practice & Health Care,* (eds S.M. Hinchcliffe, S.E. Norman & J.E. Schober) 3rd edn. Arnold, London.

Fulop, N.J., Hood, S. & Parsons, S. (1997) Does the NHS want hospital at home? *Journal of the Royal Society of Medicine,* 90, 212–15.

Green, A. (1994) The successor to patient focused care: hospital process re-engineering. *Health Summary,* 11, 6–9.

Gulland, A. (1998) Top nurse 'delighted' at new opportunities. *Nursing Times,* **94**(4), 9.

Hamilton, H., O'Byrne, M. & Nicolai, L. (1995) Central lines inserted by clinical nurse specialists. *Nursing Times,* **91**(17), 38–9.

Hoggett, P. (1996) New models of control in the public service. *Public Administration,* 74, 9–32.

Mackereth, C. (1996) Health visiting: is it a nursing matter? *Health Visitor,* **70**(4), 155–7.

Manthey, M. (1994) The patient focused approach: professional identity and the multi-skilled approach. *Journal of Nursing Administration,* **24**(10), 9–11.

McCormack, A., Fleming, D. & Charlton, J. (1995) *Morbidity statistics from general practice.* 4th National Study RCGP/OPCS. HMSO, London.

McGregor, D. (1960) *The Human Side of Enterprise.* McGraw Hill, New York.

McMahon, R. (1991) Therapeutic nursing: theory, issues and practice. In: *Nursing as Therapy,* (R. McMahon & A. Pearson). Chapman and Hall, London.

Morgan, G. & Ramirez, R. (1983) Action learning: a holographic metaphor to guide social change. *Human Relations,* 37, 1–28.

MoH (Ministry of Health) (1920) *Interim report on the future provision of medical and allied services.* The Consultative Council on Medical and Allied Services (Dawson Committee). Cmnd 693. HMSO, London.

NHSE (1997) *Personal Medical Services Pilots under the NHS (Primary Care) Act 1997.* NHS Executive, London.

NHSE (1998a) *Better health and better health care: implementing 'The New NHS' and 'Our Healthier Nation'.* HSC 1998/021. NHS Executive, London.

NHSE (1998b) *The New NHS Modern and Dependable: A National Framework for Assessing Performance.* NHS Executive, London.

NHSE (1998c) *The new NHS Modern and Dependable: Developing Primary Care Groups.* HSC 1998/139. NHS Executive, London.

NHSE (1998d) *A First Class Service: Quality in the New NHS.* NHS Executive, London.

Nolan, M.R. (1994) Geriatric nursing, an idea whose time has gone: a polemic. *Journal of Advanced Nursing,* 20, 989–96.

Pollitt, C. (1993) The struggle for quality: the case of the National Health Service. *Policy & Politics,* 21, 161–70.

Pollitt, C. (1996) Business approaches to quality improvement: why they are hard for the NHS to swallow. *Quality in Health Care,* 5, 104–10.

Porter-O'Grady, T. (1993) Patient focused care service models and nursing: perils and possibilities. *Journal of Nurse Administration,* **23**(3), 7–8, 15.

RCN (1992) *Talk Focused Hospitals of Patient Focused Care.* Royal College of Nursing, London.

Robinson, J. (1994) The problems with paradigms in a caring profession. In: *Models, Theories and Concepts*, (ed. J. Smith). Blackwell Science, Oxford.

Rowe, J. (1998) Primary opportunity. *Health Visitor*, **71**(2), 49.

Royal Commission on Medical Education (1968) *Report on 1965–1968 Cmnd 3569.* HMSO, London.

Russell, J. (1994) *A review of health promotion in primary care.* Greater London Association of Community Health Councils, London.

Starfield, B. (1992) *Primary care: concept, evaluation, and policy.* Oxford University Press, New York.

Starfield, B. (1994) Is primary care essential? *Lancet* 344, 1129–33.

Symonds, A. (1997) Ties that bind: problems with GP attachment. *Health Visitor*, **70**(2), 53–5.

Thomas, L. (1992) *A comparison of the work of qualified nurses and nursing auxiliaries in primary, team and functioning nursing wards.* Unpublished PhD thesis. University of Newcastle upon Tyne.

Walby, S. June, G. Mackay, L. & Soothill, K. (1994) *Medicine and Nursing Professions in a Changing Health Service.* Sage, London.

Index

affect
  caring as, 38–9
  nursing as, 43–5
agency nurses, 111
altruism, 8, 30, 40
apprenticeship model of training and
     education of nurses, 123, 125–6, 136
Audit Commission, 73, 76, 92
audit groups, 70
autonomous practice, professionalism and,
     6–8, 71

bank nurses, 111
bedside workers, 7
Briggs Report, 83, 88
bureaucracy, 10, 61, 164
burnout, 26

caring, 5, 8, 20, 152, 155–65
  analysis of, 36–50
     components of care, 37–41
     focusing definition, 47–50
     nursing ideals and, 41–7
     perspectives on care and caring, 36–7
  case study, 21, 22
  changing patterns of, 174–6
  context
     health policy and political, 162–5
     historical, 157–8
     organisational, 160–62
     role of, 155–7
     social and cultural, 158–60
  idealised, 21–32
  nature of, 22–8
     as affect, 38–9
     as interpersonal interaction, 39–40
     as metaphor, 24–5
     as moral imperative, 40–41, 48–9
     as therapeutic intervention, 38–9
     dichotomy, 22–3, 38
     gender and, 25–6
     holism and humanism, 23–4
  opportunities in managerial age and, 177–8
  reasons for, 28–30
     benefits for patients, 28–9
     in nursing, 30–32
     nurses' perceptions, 29–30
case management, 106–7, 110, 116
chronic illness, 90–91, 97–8, 123
class, nursing and, 83, 84, 157
clients see patients
clinical guidelines, use of, 178–9

colleges see universities and colleges
Commission for Health Improvement, 69
commissioning functions, 169–70
community (district) nursing, 7, 13, 91, 106,
     175
competence-based education, 137–8
computerisation, 67
conditions of service, 70
congestive heart failure, 91
consultation documents, 41–2
consumerism, 70–71
continuing professional development,
     114–15, 131–6
corporate image, 76
culture
  cultural context of nursing, 158–60
  cultural iatrogenesis, 9
  organisational see organisational culture of
     NHS

decision-making, participation in, 112
degree programmes, 70, 126–7
demographic changes, 89–91, 123
dichotomous nature of caring, 22–3, 38
DipHE programme, 124, 125, 127–9, 136
  fitness for purpose, 130–31
  higher education context, 129–30
district (community) nursing, 7, 13, 91, 106,
     175
doctors see medical profession
double-loop learning, 13–14, 178

education see training and education of
     nurses
elderly people, 90–91, 97–8, 116, 123
emotions, 44
empathy, 30, 44
empowerment, 9
enrolled nurses, 7
equality, 45–6
ethics see moral imperative
European Union, 4
existentialism, 37, 70

functional analysis, 137–8
functional nursing (task allocation), 103, 104,
     107–8, 109, 110, 114–15, 117, 177

gender
  caring imperative and, 25–6
  gendered nature of nursing, 5, 7, 25–6,
     44

183